Leading and Managing Veterinary Teams

Leading and Managing Veterinary Teams

The Definitive Guide to Veterinary Practice Management

Amanda L. Donnelly, DVM, MBA

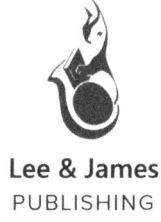

Lee & James
PUBLISHING

Leading and Managing Veterinary Teams

Copyright © 2022 by Amanda L. Donnelly

Visit the author's website at
www.amandadonnellydvm.com

ll rights reserved. No part of this publication may be reproduced or transmitted in any form or by any means, electronic or mechanical, including photocopy, recording, scanning, or any information storage and retrieval system, without permission in writing from the publisher. The forms may be reproduced for use by the person purchasing this publication but may not be sold, transferred, conveyed, or provided to any third party. For permission requests, email adonnelly@aldvet.com.

Limits of Liability/Disclaimer of Warranty

The information provided within this book is for general informational and educational purposes only. Although the author has made every effort to ensure that the information in this book was correct at press time, advances in veterinary medicine or practice management may cause information contained herein to become outdated, invalid, or subject to debate. The author makes no representations or warranties, express or implied, about the completeness, accuracy, reliability, suitability or availability with respect to the information, products, services, or related graphics contained in this book for any purpose. The author does not assume and hereby disclaims liability for errors, omissions, or any loss or damage suffered by any person as a result of the information or content in this book.

Published in the United States by Lee & James Publishing
www.leeandjamespublishing.com

First Edition

Library of Congress Control Number: 2021922486

ISBN: 978-0-578-30896-8

Printed in the United States of America

To Dad for your unconditional love and support. Your passion for learning, living life to the fullest, and helping pets and people always inspires me.

And to the loving memory of Mom and my brother, Sean, who were reunited with some amazing dogs and cats at the Rainbow Bridge.

Contents

A Note from Amanda	ix
List of Tables and Figures	xiii
Acknowledgements	xv
1 Becoming a Successful Manager	1
2 Enhancing the Hospital Culture	19
3 Recruiting and Hiring Team Members	45
4 Team Training	67
5 Enhancing and Evaluating Job Performance	91
6 Employee Retention	119
7 Communication Challenges and Solutions	139
8 Hospital Operations	165
9 Financial Management	187
10 Marketing and Client Communications	211
References	249
Appendix A: Detailed Table of Contents	259
About the Author	267

A Note from Amanda

I was 12 years old when I met Dutch, a black lab who belonged to one of my dad's best clients. Everyone at my dad's animal hospital loved Dutch. He was a handsome, affectionate, and well-mannered dog. I'll never forget how on one Sunday morning in June, my dad saved Dutch. It was one of those mornings when the humidity and heat index are high, and people don't realize their pets are susceptible to heat stroke at such an early hour. Dad and I met Dutch's owner at the hospital. Dutch was panting and couldn't walk so we all rushed him to the treatment room turning on lights as we went. I helped my father give Dutch intravenous fluids and slowly cool him down. I watched in awe as Dutch recovered and I saw the relief on his owner's face. That was one of many childhood experiences that inspired me to follow in my father's footsteps and become a veterinarian.

If you're like me, you became a veterinarian so you can heal pets and promote the human-animal bond. Or perhaps you're a manager who works in the veterinary profession because you love working with teams that help pets and people. Maybe you're a veterinary team member or have another affiliated role in veterinary medicine. You know the joy of seeing a new puppy or kitten and a client's smiling face when someone hands a pet back to them. Of course, days at a veterinary hospital aren't all full of happiness. I found that out quickly when I went into practice after veterinary school. Clients yelled at me sometimes. I found out how challenging it is to develop a great team and culture. I experienced first-hand the stress of management and leadership. As a practice leader, I made some mistakes because I didn't know any better at the time. Fortunately, over the years I learned to be a better manager and leader. I had some excellent mentors and colleagues that helped me, and I committed to ongoing learning. For me, getting an MBA was beneficial because it gave me additional knowledge in business fundamentals such as leadership, finance, and marketing. My suggestion is that you choose to continue your own learning based on your particular needs and goals.

Now as a consultant and speaker, I see and hear about the frustrations and stress practice leaders experience every day. The good news is you don't have to be worn out and worn down by management problems. You can have the empowered team you want and the culture you desire. You can have a successful practice that runs smoothly even when you aren't there. I designed *Leading and Managing Veterinary Teams* to be your go-to resource to find solutions for the common challenges you face on a weekly basis. You will discover answers to your most frequent questions and learn how to avoid common pitfalls many practice leaders face. The three major themes of this book are culture, communication, and leadership. By developing expertise in these areas, you will be in the best position to achieve practice goals and have a thriving business.

This book is for anyone involved in leading and managing veterinary teams, anyone who aspires to have such a role, or anyone who wants to learn more about veterinary practice management. I've included comprehensive, practical information to benefit all practice leaders. This includes practice owners, hospital administrators, practice managers, associate veterinarians, middle managers, and regional managers. I use the term "manager" in the text to refer to whoever is responsible for daily management and operations. If you're a practice owner, you likely have some involvement in management. Not only can this book help you hone your leadership skills and make better business decisions, it can help you understand how to best develop your managers.

The goal of this book is to provide relevant content and easy to implement action steps especially in the areas of employee communications, daily operations, and client relations. The first chapter helps you appreciate the requisite skills and knowledge every manager needs to be successful. Chapter two presents critical information you need to know to create a positive culture including how to develop a values-based organization. Chapters three through seven provide guidance on how to recruit and retain the best team members. These chapters include detailed sections on everyday concerns managers face such as lack of accountability, finding ways to improve team training, how to empower the team, and how to manage difficult employee communications.

I've also included chapters on hospital operations, financial management, and marketing with an emphasis on how these areas of management relate to your team. In chapter eight, you'll gain an understanding of how to find the best ways to increase operational efficiency. Since practices can't survive without being profitable, chapter nine outlines the most important aspects of financial management and which key performance indicators every practice should monitor. And finally, chapter ten on marketing and client communications presents specific actions to take to thrive in today's competitive marketplace. The primary focus of this chapter is how to train the team to enhance client engagement, build client loyalty, and increase compliance by using specific communication skills.

A Note from Amanda

When I was in my second year of veterinary school, I lost my 14-year-old Siamese cat to renal failure. My mom was determined to find me a Siamese kitten which was a tall order considering it was December. Right after Christmas, amazingly, she found a 13-week-old, male, seal-point Siamese in a neighborhood not too far away. We got in the car to go home with my mom ready to drive and me in the passenger seat holding the kitten. She looked over, smiled, and said, "Let's name him "Peppermint" because he's a life saver!"

I believe our pets are like life savers and I can't imagine life without mine. My hope is that you will remember how valuable your career is even on those tough days. I hope the guidance, concepts, and solutions in this book will help decrease your stress and the difficulties associated with leadership and management so you can continue to support your team and serve our great profession. What you do makes a difference in the lives of pet owners and helps more pets get care they deserve.

I'm proud to be a part of the veterinary profession and grateful for all the opportunities I've had to work with team members. I commend you for your dedication to pets and people. I'm personally honored to share this journey of learning and lifelong love of pets together with you.

Amanda L. Donnelly, DVM, MBA

List of Tables

Table 1.1	Characteristics of Reactive Leaders vs. Proactive Leaders
Table 1.2	Time Management Strategies
Table 1.3	Truths and Myths about Managing Up
Table 1.4	Leadership Actions That Build or Break Down Trust
Table 3.1	What to Include in Job Ads
Table 3.2	Recruitment Strategies Best Practices
Table 3.3	Legal vs. Illegal Interview Questions
Table 3.4	Effective Interview Questions
Table 5.1	Effective Delegation Process
Table 5.2	Characteristics of Effective vs. Ineffective Feedback
Table 5.3	Lack of Accountability: Causes and Characteristics
Table 5.4	Communication Process for Accountability Meetings
Table 6.1	Retention Strategies
Table 7.1	Steps to Facilitate Conflict Resolution Meetings
Table 8.1	Causes of Operational Inefficiency
Table 9.1	Assessing Causes of High Support Staff Payroll
Table 10.1	Client Acquisition Strategies

List of Figures

Figure 2.1	Example Veterinary Practice SWOT Analysis
Figure 2.2	Team Worksheet for Developing Core Values *
Figure 2.3	Strategic Planning Worksheet *
Figure 2.4	Race and Ethnicity in Veterinary Medicine
Figure 4.1	New Hire Orientation Checklist *
Figure 4.2	New Hire Survey *
Figure 4.3	Technician/Assistant On-boarding Checklist *
Figure 4.4	Technician/Assistant Training Checklist *
Figure 4.5	Training Team Roles *
Figure 4.6	Checklist to Implement an Effective Training Program *
Figure 5.1	How Often Employees Say They Receive Feedback from Their Managers
Figure 5.2	Performance Improvement Plan (PIP) *
Figure 6.1	Benefits of High Employee Engagement
Figure 6.2	What Gen Z Wants in the Workplace
Figure 6.3	Employee Developmental Plan *
Figure 7.1	Project Team Roles and Responsibilities *
Figure 8.1	Protocol Template *
Figure 8.2	SOP Template *
Figure 8.3	Job Description Meeting Facilitator *
Figure 9.1	How to Grow Practice Revenue *
Figure 10.1	Client Communications Team Training Exercises *
Figure 10.2	Social Media Usage by Generation
Figure 10.3	Facebook Usage by Generation

*Denotes form available to download at www.amandadonnellydvm.com

Acknowledgements

Writing this book would not have been possible without the influence and help of some special people in my life.

First I must express my profound gratitude to my dad who showed me the joy and fulfillment of a career in veterinary medicine which is why I followed in his footsteps. Thank you for always encouraging me and showing me the value of connecting with clients to help pets get the care they deserve.

To my mom because her love of all animals, and in particular her passion for dogs, inspired both Dad and me to become a veterinarian. She taught me how to stay organized and that hard work helps you reach your goals. It was my mom who encouraged me to join the high school speech and debate team because she knew I needed an outlet for all my words. Excelling at extemporaneous speaking and debate laid the foundation for me to become a professional speaker.

A special appreciation goes to my niece, Rachel Donnelly-Mason, for giving me a somewhat funny, practical book on how to write better and more efficiently. I'm also grateful for all the times you've patiently listened to me, made me laugh, shared your knowledge, and brightened my day with your generosity and marvelous smile.

My deepest thanks to my amazing friend, Freddie Tezak, who has given me invaluable business advice and insight that has helped me succeed in countless ways. I'm grateful for your generosity, unwavering support, and that you remind me to celebrate my success. I can't imagine not having you as my person.

To my dear friend, Dr. Sam Romano, I appreciate you sharing your knowledge on leadership, culture, and communications. Thank you for your keen insight and always asking thoughtful questions. You've helped me through some tough times and been one of my biggest cheerleaders. Every time we talk, I'm inspired to learn more and keep following my dreams.

To Dr. Peter Weinstein, I want to extend my gratitude for your wisdom and friendship. You've always been willing to listen and offer practical advice on how to get past the bumps in the road. Thanks to you, I'm looking through the front windshield and staying focused on my priorities.

I also want to recognize Dr. Ron Cott who is an incredibly gracious mentor and friend. Thank you for your kindness and always supporting me. Your commitment to family, friends, clients, colleagues, students, and our profession knows no bounds.

Thank you to all the practice owners, managers, and team members who've told me their stories, asked for advice, shared their challenges, and implemented positive change. I'm grateful that I have the opportunity to work with such incredible veterinary teams that work so hard to enhance the human-pet bond.

And lastly, thank you to all my family, friends, and colleagues who have supported me in my journey.

CHAPTER 1

Becoming a Successful Manager

Regardless of their level of education, experience, or business skills, people motivated to learn and grow are the most likely to excel in leadership and management roles. You may be a practice manager reading this book to learn as much as you can to fully contribute to your practice. Or you may be a practice owner who wants to learn more about management and how to best work with your manager to enhance the success of your business. Perhaps you were recently promoted into a management role and feel you need to develop the requisite skills and knowledge to be a successful manager. Maybe you have credentials and management experience in another industry but lack knowledge about the veterinary industry. On the other hand, you may be a veterinary manager with extensive knowledge and expertise who is reading this book to learn anything you can to optimize your team's performance. This chapter outlines areas of focus for anyone in a management role that wants to be successful. No matter what your background is, think about your development and what actions you want to take to be enhance your success.

DEFINING SUCCESS

What does it mean to be a successful manager? Or if you're an experienced manager, a better question to ask yourself might be, "How can I be *more* successful in my job?" People tend to have different answers about what it means to be successful. Some view their success as it relates to helping other people. Others measure success based on the outcome of each day or week. Managers may define success based on personal feelings about their job performance. Practice owners may consider their managers successful if clients and the team are happy. While these are all valid perspectives, they are arbitrary assessments. Rather than only using subjective criteria, it's wise to view success from a business perspective and whether the manager is contributing to the success of the practice. Successful managers accomplish daily work assignments, build positive cultures, achieve assigned goals, and enhance the practice's growth and profitability.

It is worth noting that your definition of success needs to align with the owners of the business. Discussing what it means to be a successful manger helps both parties avoid breakdowns in communication and misunderstandings which could affect your job satisfaction as well as your job security.

BEING PROACTIVE VS. REACTIVE

Becoming a successful manager begins by developing a proactive versus a reactive approach to the business. Reactive managers tend to only focus on what must get done each day and only deal with conflict or problems when they have to. Conversely, proactive managers resist complacency; they spend time on activities that help achieve goals and improve the business. There will be days when even the most proactive manager has to react to solve pressing problems and address challenges. But proactive managers know how to get back on track after a hectic day or month. They constantly strive to better themselves and take action to make the business more successful. While proactive managers spend time on planning and business development, this time pays off because it increases their efficiency and productivity. (See Table 1.1 for characteristics of reactive and proactive managers.)

Table 1.1: Characteristics of Reactive Managers vs. Proactive Managers

Reactive Managers	Proactive Managers
Are task oriented	Are results oriented
Focus on short-term goals	Focus on short and long-term goals
Have a to-do list that never gets done	Complete action steps on time to reach goals
Fail to spend sufficient time on planning	Engage in strategic planning
Don't always develop systems	Put systems in place
Are always putting out fires	Don't routinely have to deal with crises
Are conflict averse	Deal with conflict when it arises
Slow to make decisions	Make decisions without delays
Neglect team development	Focus on building trust with the team and developing team members

ESTABLISHING JOB EXPECTATIONS

Being an effective manager begins with your job description. However, it's not uncommon for everyone in the practice to have a job description except the manager. How can you be successful without a clearly defined job description? It's an essential communication tool that provides you and your employer with a clear understanding of what job duties you were hired to perform and your areas of responsibilities. The major areas of responsibility for managers may include human resource management, operations, marketing, and financial management. Another problem that happens all too often is that managers end up with a generic job description that details various job duties for an office manager or a practice manager, but nobody tailored it to specify the job duties and job roles for the person currently filling the position at the hospital.

Once you have a job description, review it for accuracy. Do you currently fulfill the job duties and roles as outlined in the job description or does the document need to be modified? Remember your job description should include all your job duties. For example, a veterinary technician or assistant who is a supervisor, should have a job description for their primary position that includes a section outlining all their management job duties. Likewise, if you're a manager that used to fulfill job duties as a client service representative or a member of the technical team, then your job description needs to clarify whether you still have responsibilities in these departments.

The next step is to make sure your job description includes job expectations. This is one of the most critical yet overlooked aspects of job descriptions. Job expectations provide clarity on how you will do your job and your level of responsibility. The value of including these specifics cannot be overstated. Written job expectations help employees and bosses alike avoid assumptions which could lead to hurt feelings, issues with job satisfaction, and problems with job performance. Here are examples of job expectations you may want to include in your job description:

- The expected dress code
- Work schedule including expected arrival time for shifts, which days of the week are workdays, expected number of hours per week, ability to work overtime or stay late, and whether you can ever work from home
- Availability to team members when not scheduled to work or when the practice is closed
- Ability to lift a specific amount of weight or stand for a specified time period

- What time will be allotted for management job duties (this is important for employees whose primary job role is not in management)
- For managers with multiple job roles, how many hours will be spent working "on the floor" and how many hours will be spent doing managerial duties
- Job priorities
- Attendance at marketing functions
- Attendance at outside continuing education programs
- Authority and autonomy; e. g., Do you have permission to hire and terminate employees without approval? Can you make purchases up to a specific amount without seeking approval? Are you authorized to fire clients who demonstrate unacceptable behavior?

Setting job expectations also includes defining accountability for outcomes and job performance. For example, are you accountable for ensuring hospital expenses stay within budget? If your job description states "Maintain major practice expense categories within target goals" you and your boss should agree on appropriate expectations and action steps to fulfill this job responsibility. Otherwise, the job description is just words on paper and in reality, you may or may not be accountable for controlling expenses. Likewise, there may not be a plan or timeline in place to respond to increases in expense categories if they occur.

Job descriptions and job expectations serve as the foundation for performance appraisals. Your job performance evaluation should assess whether you're successfully completing your assigned job duties, meeting expectations, accomplishing goals, and making positive contributions to the practice. Just like every other team member in the practice, managers benefit from having regular reviews with their boss. Sometimes managers are so busy completing employee reviews they neglect to schedule their own review. Don't make this mistake. At a minimum, sit down annually with your supervisor for a formal job performance evaluation that is supported with written documentation. This ensures you have an opportunity to receive feedback on your job performance, discuss your development, review progress on goals, and establish future plans.

ENHANCING PRODUCTIVITY

When considering your productivity, think about both the quality and quantity of your work. Performing quality work is paramount but if you don't consistently complete assignments or projects in a timely manner, the business may suffer. The keys to being productive are both proficiency and efficiency which isn't always easy. For example, consider the employee review process. Effective employee reviews should be comprehensive, objective, and thoughtful. Team members should walk away knowing how they're doing, where they need to improve, and defined action steps to take to meet their goals. If this describes your review process, then you are proficient in this area of management. But are you efficient? Do you schedule employee reviews on time? Efficient managers implement a process that ensures employee reviews happen when they are supposed to so team members can gain valuable feedback they need to enhance their job performance.

Being productive equates to being effective with time management. Veterinary practice managers often struggle with time management due to the high demands of their jobs. Managers are frequently pulled in different directions to respond to the needs of clients, team members, and business owners all the while striving to keep the practice running smoothly. It can be difficult to balance completing daily work duties with activities to reach hospital goals. As a starting point, recognize that no one can manage time. You have the same reasonable number of hours each week to complete job-related activities. Rather than thinking about how to manage time, focus on *how* you spend your time. In his book, *Leadership Isn't for Cowards*, Mike Staver writes that time management is "……about getting the highest rate of return on the *energy* you invest on a daily basis." He also recommends leaders spend time on high-gain activities.[1] These are the activities that done consistently will have the greatest impact on the organization.

Stephen R. Covey's book, *The Seven Habits of Highly Successful People*, also points out the importance of engaging in activities that drive the success of your business. He writes, "…. the best thinking in the area of time management can be captured in a single phrase: *Organize and execute around priorities*." He also states that "……"time management" is really a misnomer—the challenge is not to manage time, but to manage ourselves."[2] Covey presented The Time Management Matrix in his book which outlines the four ways people spend time. In his model, activities are either important or not important and urgent or not urgent. He identified the importance of spending time on not urgent but important tasks because these activities focus on the mission, values, and goals of the business. Examples of important work activities that aren't urgent include time spent on team training and developing programs for team well-being.

Clearly, one of the keys to being a successful manager is to prioritize job duties and stay focused on action steps to achieve goals. To avoid the pitfall of becoming a reactive manager, be sure to define both short and long-term goals. Of course, you may set a daily schedule for how much you want to accomplish only to find your work is derailed if urgent problems arise such as the need to talk to an upset client or handle a computer software issue. These situations are usually unavoidable. But remember that even if you don't meet your daily goal, you can still hopefully attain your weekly goal.

Setting weekly objectives is an excellent way to make progress on project work, personal development, or activities to attain hospital goals. One of the biggest challenges in achieving some business goals is that they can seem overwhelming. Executing a strategic marketing plan, for example, requires multiple action steps by the leadership team. Likewise, efforts to enhance employee engagement and empowerment may seem daunting since this is a broad goal. Creating an organized process to tackle large projects is helpful for anyone responsible for planning and coordinating these types of activities. Establishing weekly targets helps to maintain focus and break down the project into all the incremental action steps necessary to accomplish the business goal.

Now that you understand the importance of determining *how* you spend time at work, you may still need to identify time management strategies to maximize your productivity. Try several approaches, if necessary, to find the ones that work best for you. (See Table 1.2 for a summary of proven time management strategies.) There are a variety of time management strategies that can help you stay focused on priorities and goals including the following:

- Determine when you have the most energy as this is your time to be the most productive. This may be early in the morning or on certain days of the week.
- Set time blocks for specific project and goal work. Avoid multi-tasking as this can lead to working on many projects but never finishing anything. Many managers find it helpful to close their office door for a few hours and put up a sign alerting the team they're unavailable unless someone has an urgent need. This strategy only works well if you communicate with the team why you need designated time to complete work and coach employees to problem-solve if they interrupt with non-urgent needs.
- Avoid distractions when doing project work; avoid working in close proximity to others, turn off unnecessary or non-urgent notifications on your cell phone or computer, limit time spent on the internet and social media.
- Recognize that you cannot do it all. Managers are more productive if they effectively delegate and empower their team. (For more information, see Chapter 5 on Enhancing and Evaluating Job Performance and Chapter 6 on Employee Retention.) Successful managers work with their practice owners to seek assistance

when needed. For example, you may need to outsource activities related to digital marketing, HR compliance, and bookkeeping.

- Use time tracking and planning tools such as planners, time management apps, and progress trackers. Many people find it helpful to use digital tools or spreadsheets for time tracking as a way to increase efficiency and identify time wasters.

Table 1.2: Time Management Strategies

Strategy	Description
Limit time spent on email and the internet	<ul><li>Review email 2-3 times/day at a designated time; rely on pop-up notifications for urgent matters</li><li>Avoid the temptation to surf the net, watch videos, check social media, or read news</li><li>Unsubscribe from e-newsletters that aren't high value, or you never read</li></ul>
Prioritize job duties	<ul><li>Spend time at the beginning of the day on the most important, high-value job tasks</li></ul>
Set weekly goals	<ul><li>Outline weekly goals at the beginning of the week</li></ul>
Plan ahead	<ul><li>Plan the next day before leaving work</li><li>Keep a separate list of non-urgent activities and projects</li></ul>
Organize daily activities	<ul><li>Time block job tasks on a daily planner</li><li>Avoid interruptions and complete work unless there is an urgent problem</li></ul>
Be willing to say no	<ul><li>Set boundaries and say no to activities that aren't important or time sensitive</li><li>Schedule time at a later date for non-urgent interruptions</li></ul>
Keep track of interruptions	<ul><li>Look for opportunities to delegate job duties and train team members so they can act without seeking direction or approval</li></ul>

Table 1.2: Time Management Strategies (continued)

Strategy	Description
Take breaks	- Take short 5-15 minutes breaks every 1-2 hours - Move or walk around; take a break from computer work
Conduct time audits	- Periodically track time spent on job duties each week and evaluate what's working well and what's not working well

HONING COMMUNICATION SKILLS

Perhaps the single most important quality of a successful manager is the ability to effectively communicate with the team. Enhancing communication skills is a vital life skill that helps people connect, build rapport, and develop stronger relationships. If you've ever thought about how you communicate and said, "I can't change who I am!" or "That's just how I communicate", then think again. Everyone can learn how to improve their communications.

Active Listening

Active listening is defined as the process of thoughtfully listening to understand the message of another person. With active listening, people mindfully focus on what is being said rather than what their response will be to the person talking.[3] Active listening is a valuable skill for managers who want to learn relevant information, gain feedback, and ensure employees feel heard. The skill of active listening takes practice. Use the following techniques to improve your active listening skills.

- Be mindful of using non-verbal communications that conveys your interest in the other person. Maintain eye contact, lean in slightly and nod occasionally to indicate you're listening.
- Don't interrupt; let the other person complete a thought before asking questions.
- Pause for a few seconds after the other person stops talking. This shows respect and gives you an opportunity to think before speaking.

Transparent Communication

Transparent communication in the workplace refers to the open and honest sharing of information across all teams. Practices that have cultures with transparent communication encourage everyone to speak candidly and respectfully. Successful managers build trust by keeping everyone on the team informed even if it is to say, "We haven't made a decision yet, but this is the latest update." Being transparent also means being willing to be vulnerable and own up to mistakes. When appropriate, you might say a phrase such as "I see that this didn't go well, and I made a mistake."

Problems arise if practice owners or managers feel information should only be shared on a "need to know basis." Inevitably, in this situation team members perceive management isn't being straightforward and honest which results in a breakdown of trust. Employees don't like being kept in the dark and they definitely don't like surprises. Without transparent communication, people tend to gossip or keep secrets, and the grapevine takes over as a means of communication in the hospital.

Transparency is particularly important during times of change. During the recession of 2008 and the COVID-19 pandemic crisis that started in 2020, managers who kept their teams apprised of how the business was doing built trust. As a manager, you want to be transparent about possible changes such as staff shortages, for example, while at the same time conveying confident messages of hope and resilience. In her book, *Dare to Lead*, Brené Brown speaks to the value of transparency as she shares her research on vulnerability and leadership. Her work shows the need for successful leaders to demonstrate empathy and be willing to have courageous conversations with their teams.[4]

Asking Good Questions

Building the habit of asking good questions is an invaluable communication skill. Similar to active listening, asking questions demonstrates your interest in team members and helps them feel heard. You can ask questions simply to create dialogue and build rapport. This includes questions such as "Did you do anything interesting or fun this weekend?", "Tell me how your daughter did at her piano recital", and "What are your favorite activities outside of work?" Questions are also a great way to solicit ideas from team members. You could ask "How do you think we can provide better training for new hires?", "What ideas do you have to get more involved in community events?", and "Tell me more about your ideas to improve our Facebook page."

Asking questions helps you gain relevant information and avoid assumptions because questions invite team members to share their thoughts, feedback, and feelings.

This is particularly important when talking to team members about their job performance and when facilitating conflict resolution meetings. For example, you can avoid assumptions about the motivations behind an employee's behavior by asking "What is your perspective on what happened?" or "Tell me how you came to that decision." The benefit of taking time to ask questions and listen to the answers, is to gain a better understanding of employees. You can learn more about what motivates team members, their perspectives and discover what they need to do their job better.

Setting Boundaries

Managers need to be available to team members who ask for relevant information, support, feedback, and advice. However, managers may unwittingly become the go-to resource for employees who want to vent, complain, and dump their problems onto someone else to solve. To avoid this scenario, set healthy boundaries with team members. This may be difficult for managers who are friends with their co-workers or those who feel they need to jump in to help employees solve their personal problems. (To learn more about coaching employees who consistently complain, see Chapter 7 on Communication Challenges and Solutions.)

It's important to clearly communicate boundaries to the team. Some boundaries are set forth in the employee handbook. This includes the hospital code of conduct, anti-discrimination, anti-harassment and diversity and inclusion policies. Here are a few examples of other boundaries managers may want to establish with employees:

- The need to distinguish between professional and personal relationships. While this might not always be realistic, ideally practice managers should limit socializing with co-workers to work-related events and avoid connecting with co-workers on social media.
- When it is and is not acceptable to text, email or call after work hours.
- Avoiding oversharing of personal information. Managers can promote a positive, family-oriented culture but also maintain professional relationships. They may need to let team members know they aren't an appropriate sounding board to hear everything about an employee's family drama, financial woes, or personal relationships.

MANAGING UP

The terminology "managing up" or "managing your boss" has many definitions and isn't always clearly understood. Thomas J. Zuber, MD and Erika H. James, PhD, both professors at Emory University, define managing up as "the process of consciously working with your boss to obtain the best possible results for you, your boss and your organization."[5] Managing up doesn't mean you are "kissing up" or trying to manipulate your boss. It's about cultivating a positive working relationship that allows you to be a more effective manager and advance your career while also helping your boss.[6] (See Table 1.3 for a summary of what is and is not managing up.)

There are different types of practice owner-manager relationships. You may report to the sole owner of the business, multiple owners, a hospital administrator, a board of directors, the medical director, or a regional manager if a corporation owns your practice. Regardless of who owns the business, the process of managing up is the same. But you will have a more nuanced approach if the business has multiple owners. In these instances, be sure to establish who you report to and the process for decision-making. Let's say, for example, two partners own your practice. You may report weekly to one for HR management decisions and the other for decisions related to financial management. The three of you may meet monthly to discuss all aspects of management and progress toward achieving hospital goals.

Establishing open lines of communication is critical to any relationship. To successfully manage up, determine what type of communication works best for your boss. Do they prefer texts, emails, digital platforms, or face-to-face meetings? What is their preferred time of day to meet? Regardless of the method of communication, managers and practice owners need to meet regularly to discuss hospital management and operations. When asked about when they meet with their boss, managers frequently report they just talk to them every day. This way of communicating isn't inherently problematic, but it isn't efficient. Inevitably, managers find themselves having rushed and disorganized conversations that don't allow sufficient time to discuss hospital business. A much better approach is to schedule meetings for a specific time and day of the week. During this meeting, managers can discuss relevant issues and confirm their weekly goals which helps them be more productive.

Seeking to understand your boss is one of the best ways to develop a productive working relationship. Take time to consider their business perspectives, work style, leaderships traits, and communication preferences. Observe how they respond to pressure and workplace stresses. If you have a long-standing relationship with your boss or the owner of the practice, take a step back and evaluate what works well in your relationship and identify when you've both experienced some bumps in the road. Regardless of how long you've known your boss, ask questions to gain a better understanding of what motivates them, their personal aspirations, and their professional goals; remember their answers may change over time.

Have you ever tried to implement positive changes only to meet resistance from whoever you report to? This is when understanding the business owner's motivators and goals helps you become a more successful manager. If money is a primary motivator for your practice owner, for example, then communicate how a proposed change will increase revenues, make the business more competitive, or ultimately enhance profitability. Be prepared to explain the return on investment for any proposed expenditures. If the business owner is concerned about team morale, show them how your plans for change will create a better work environment and enhance employee retention.

To successfully manage up, it's imperative to understand and be able to adapt to the communication style of your supervisor. This can help you prepare for meetings and avoid frustrating conversations. Are they reserved, calm, long-winded, moody, easily stressed, indecisive, easy-going, or conflict avoidant? Do they like to talk through problems, or do they need time to process information? Does your boss like direct recommendations or prefer having multiple options to evaluate? This may affect whether you need one or more meetings to finalize decisions. If you know your supervisor doesn't like strong suggestions, you can use softer language such as "We might try this" or "Have you thought about this approach?"

Managing up also entails anticipating the needs of your boss and taking action to make their job easier or less stressful. In large part, you do this simply by doing your job well but also by thinking ahead. For example, you could proactively seek cost savings for the business by evaluating current digital marketing initiatives and vendor relationships. Perhaps you could identify ways to help streamline client communications for the doctors. Be sure to propose solutions to problems when discussing hospital challenges. Offer suggestions that demonstrate you've given the problem some thought and considered ways to improve operations. Even better, let your bosses know how you can help implement the solutions.

People who successfully manage up take responsibility to make their relationship with their supervisor work even if they have a difficult boss. If you have a challenging relationship with whoever you report to, strive to demonstrate patience, and stay in control of your emotions. Be honest and ask for what you need. You could say, "I'm feeling discounted and unappreciated. I'm here to help you and the practice. I'd like to discuss how I can best do that as well as what I need to do my job." Remember that being flexible and adapting to the communication style of your boss doesn't mean tolerating unacceptable behavior.

Table 1.3: Truths and Myths about Managing Up

Truths about Managing Up	Myths about Managing Up
Seek to understand your boss	Gain favor by sucking up to your boss
Clarify job expectations and the flow of communication with all business owners	Only communicate with the practice owner who you think really likes you
Adapt your communication style to that of your boss	Communicate just like your boss
Ask questions to better understand your boss and their needs	Avoid rocking the boat and just listen to your boss
Strive to anticipate your boss's needs; make their job easier and less stressful	Agree to take on all requested job duties and assignments
Present solutions to problems	Ask for direction before taking action
Promote honest, transparent communication	Tell your boss what they want to hear
Be willing to express your thoughts and feelings	Keep your feelings to yourself
Communicate relevant team feedback	Protect your boss from negative team feedback
Call out behavior that violates core values	Tolerate bad behavior because that's part of the job

LEADERSHIP DEVELOPMENT

Management can be defined as the "process of working with and through others to achieve organizational objectives in a changing environment."[7] Leadership can be defined as the "process of influencing, inspiring and guiding others to participate in a common effort."[8] Every manager needs excellent leadership skills to be successful. While some individuals may have natural talent in this area, everyone can benefit from leadership development. Successful managers recognize that becoming an effective leader isn't a destination but rather it is a lifelong process of striving to be the best leader possible for your team.

Leadership Roles and Building Trust

Regardless of job title, one of the most significant leadership roles is to consistently model the behavior desired from the rest of the team. As leaders in the practice, the actions of managers are often scrutinized by other employees. For example, team members notice if managers are tardy or never stay late. Managers frequently have flexible schedules especially if they're on salary, and they may not have to clock in for work. But if the team has been told the manager is supposed to work 8am to 5pm, the perception is they're late if they don't arrive by 8am. Likewise, if managers never stay late to help the team, the perception is they're asking something of employees they're unwilling to do themselves. Managers need to always be mindful of the message conveyed by their behavior. (See Table 1.4 for leadership actions that build or break down trust.)

Another critical leadership role is to build trust with the team. There are several characteristics of leaders that help to build trust with employees and develop a more productive team. Here are 4 leadership qualities that have been proven to build trust.[9]

Clarity

One of the most overlooked aspects of being a trusted leader is to clearly establish the vision, core values and goals of the practice. Practice owners and managers should work together to clearly articulate these aspects of the business to employees. When team members know and understand the vision, values, and goals of the practice, it's easier for them to focus on their role in the success of the business. This strategic planning process is covered in more detail in the next chapter.

Competency

If team members don't feel practice leaders are competent, teamwork and a commitment to quality work may start to suffer. This isn't to say trusted leaders must be perfect or excel in every skill applicable to the job. But they do need to demonstrate both proficiency and efficiency with their job duties. Managers can enhance their competencies by being committed to continuous learning.

Caring

Caring leaders make authentic connections with their team which helps build trust. Managers don't need to be everyone's best friend or win favor with employees by providing freebies. Instead, the goal is to create a supportive, positive environment where people look forward to coming to work. One way to easily show you care is to offer regular praise and appreciation to team members. Another is to provide opportunities for growth. Budgetary constraints aren't a barrier for these initiatives because personal thank-you cards, and in-house mentoring or training isn't costly. Don't forget that caring extends to the clients and community. Managers also build trust with the team when they demonstrate how much they care about patients, clients, and the surrounding community.

Table 1.4: Leadership Actions That Build or Break Down Trust

Actions That Build Trust	Actions That Break Down Trust
Communicate vision and mission	Lack of clarity about vision and mission
Following through with promises	Failure to follow-up on promised action
Following established hospital policies and protocols	Lack of adherence to policies and protocols
Being on time to work and meetings	Being late for appointments or meetings
Adhering to all client service standards	Inconsistent adherence to service standards
Maintaining a positive outlook	Demonstrating negativity or mood swings
Treating all team members the same	Showing favoritism towards some employees
Praise and recognition towards all team members	Lack of praise and recognition or only recognizing a few team members
Always adhering to core values of business	Violating core values of business
Communicating clear goals	Lack of communication about hospital goals
Negative feedback in private	Negative feedback in public
Honest, straightforward communication	Lack of transparent communication
Commitment to diversity and inclusion	Failure to promote diversity and inclusion
Establishing clear expectations	Expectations unclear
Solicit and listen to employee feedback	Failure to listen to or solicit feedback

Consistency

Businesses need to have policies and procedures that are both consistent and fair. Employees want stability, transparency, and a fair workplace. Trust breaks down if the rules are constantly changing or people perceive that favoritism exists. To create a consistent work environment and build trust, establish standards and protocols that the entire team must adhere to. Other ways trusted leaders commit to consistency is to avoid favoritism, follow through with action when promises or assurances are made, and model the behavior they want from the rest of the team.

Identify Strengths and Weaknesses

To become a better leader, reflect on your strengths and weaknesses so you can identify areas of opportunity to hone leadership skills. What are you good at? Where do you need to improve? And most importantly, how do you decide? It's not unusual for people to arrive at false conclusions or have blind spots when evaluating their strengths and weaknesses. It's also easy to become complacent in answering these questions once people become established in their careers. It's human nature to be so focused on doing your job that you neglect to spend time on how to do it better. Be mindful of the concept that sometimes "we don't know what we don't know."

When assessing your strengths and weaknesses, take care to scrutinize any labels others have given you or that you've told yourself. Maybe you've been told you are a "procrastinator", "aren't good with numbers", "a people pleaser" or you "aren't creative". Ask yourself the question, "What's the evidence this label is accurate?" For example, you may not be artistic but that doesn't mean you aren't creative. You may have excellent creative-thinking and problem-solving skills. Likewise, you may feel you procrastinate but you never miss a deadline. When labeling yourself, avoid the pitfall of excusing any less than desirable behavior or habits you have by saying "Well, this is just who I am!"

Think about your successes and failures. What has worked well for you to develop job skills and build relationships? Where have you struggled the most? In addition to your own reflection, ask for feedback from people you trust. This may include colleagues, mentors, friends, family, and your boss. When soliciting feedback, actively listen and avoid any temptation to argue about the feedback or defend yourself. And ask questions to learn more. You can ask "Tell me more about that" or "Please give me some examples so I can better understand."

Personality Testing and Assessment Tools

There are a variety of assessments you can use to identify your strengths, behavioral traits, and areas for development. There is no perfect test or a right and wrong outcome. Rather these tools simply help with self-discovery, and they provide a better understanding of how you interact with others and the world. The two most popular personality tests include the Myers-Briggs Type Indicator, or MBTI, and the DISC Assessment. Both are frequently used to help people increase their personal and professional success. Another tool is the Gallup Clifton Strengths Assessment (formerly Clifton StrengthsFinder), which they report is used by millions of people to discover their natural talents so they can focus on what they do best.[10]

A different assessment is offered by the Judgment Index™ which focuses on how people make decisions. The company explains it is not a personality test and promotes the Judgement Index as the only measurement tool that focuses on a person's values when making decisions. It can be used to assist individuals and teams in their development with the goal of improving productivity as well as personal well-being.[11]

Regardless of which tests you use, consider having all members of the team take the assessment so everyone can learn how to leverage their strengths and communicate better with each other in the workplace. Remember, any assessment tool is only as good as what you do with the results. Create a plan to implement action steps that lead to enhanced productivity, better leadership, and further career development.

Professional Development

There are many resources available to help you gain knowledge, competence, skills, and expertise. You can read business articles and books, attend continuing education meetings and workshops, and take college classes in topics such as accounting. You can join mastermind groups, hire a coach, seek out a mentor or accountability partner, and work with veterinary management consultants. Professional development resources also include business leadership or networking groups in your community as well as organizations such as the Chamber of Commerce and Toastmasters.

Another resource for managers is to join professional organizations within the veterinary industry and the business community. Here are some organizations for managers to know about:

American Veterinary Medical Association (AVMA): You must be a veterinarian to join AVMA. Managers can access the resources provided by AVMA through the membership of the owner veterinarian of the practice or one of the associate veterinarians. The organization puts out a journal twice monthly that includes relevant industry news. AVMA holds an Annual Convention that includes sessions on practice management and professional development, hosts a Veterinary Leadership Conference and an Economic Summit, and has a digital education platform named AVMA Axon. The AVMA website has resources and tools in the areas of well-being, personal finance, animal health and welfare, public health, and practice management.[12]

American Animal Hospital Association (AAHA): As an organization, AAHA accredits veterinary practices in the United States and Canada. Accredited practices must meet stringent quality standards. AAHA has numerous publications and educational resources for managers in the areas of veterinary leadership and management.[13]

Veterinary Hospital Managers Association (VHMA): VHMA founded the Certified Veterinary Practice Manager (CVPM) certification program which is recognized as the highest level of credential for veterinary practice managers. VHMA members have access to management tools and publications, webinars, continuing education meetings, and an active member connect forum for managers to communicate about relevant business and management topics.[14]

Society for Human Resource Management (SHRM): SHRM offers members access to a wealth of information in the way of articles, sample tools and documents, business solutions, and certification programs. SHRM is an excellent resource for managers seeking information about HR compliance.[15]

SUMMARY

As you reflect on this chapter, you probably recognize that being successful in your career requires action. You can take action to gain more knowledge, learn new skills, become more proficient in specific areas of management or practice communication skills. Even in you have years of experience, there is always an opportunity to learn and grow. Successful people know the value of continuous learning both personally and professionally. Sometimes busy managers only focus on helping their boss and team members, so they neglect their own development. Before you dive into the rest of this book, take time to think about what you would like to do to be more successful. Write down the top three areas you want to work on to be more effective and productive in your job. Then commit to at least one action you *will* take in the next 30 days to help you achieve your goal(s). In the chapters ahead, you will learn how to enhance the practice culture and develop your team. Ultimately, your success depends on your ability to take action not only for the practice but for your own development as well.

CHAPTER 2

Enhancing the Hospital Culture

The culture of a business refers to the beliefs, values, behaviors, and shared experiences of the employees. The word "norms" is often used when defining culture to describe the typical patterns of behavior for a group. Cultures are typically viewed positively or negatively depending on the actions of everyone in the business. You've likely heard team members who either say "This is how we do it" or "That's *not* how we do things here." Depending on the context of the conversation, these statements can have a favorable or unfavorable connotation about the culture of the business. Saying "That's not how we do it here", for example, may imply employees aren't open to new ideas. On the other hand, telling a new hire, "This is how we do it here" may be referring to positive values of the organization.

When contemplating business culture, consider the reality of your *current* culture. What aspects of your practice culture come to mind? Are you happy with your culture? What picture do you see when thinking about your team as they go about their work? How would team members describe your culture? What would clients say if you asked them to describe your culture? These are important questions to ponder if you want to improve your hospital culture. Bear in mind, it's the collective actions of both practice leaders and the rest of the team that define the culture.

As you read this chapter, think about your *desired* culture and what you'd like to accomplish to enhance the culture. Is there something you want to change? Have you identified some unacceptable or unfavorable behaviors in your organization? Are you concerned about aspects of your culture that don't align with your values? Or do you simply want to continue the success you've already achieved in developing your desired culture?

The long-term success of any business is tied to culture. Without a positive culture, most practices won't attain their desired high levels of team satisfaction, employee retention, productivity, patient care, client service, growth, and profitability. But positive cultures don't just happen. Thoughtful planning helps leaders get the culture they want. In the rest of this chapter, you will read about activities and planning that are essential to having a healthy, positive culture.

STRATEGIC PLANNING

Strategic planning can be defined as the process by which business leaders determine what actions will most likely result in superior performance for the company so it can be profitable and maintain a competitive advantage in the marketplace. The strategic planning process typically involves developing the mission, vision, and values of the company, completing a SWOT analysis, and formulating goals for the business.[1] An overview of these activities is outlined in the following sections. (See Figure 2.3 for a strategic planning worksheet.)

Here's another way to think of strategic planning; it is a process of defining where the business is now, where it wants to go, and how it will get there. When viewed this way, it becomes clear how strategic planning is closely related to culture because without the collective efforts of the team, a business can't achieve its goals. Moreover, productive, engaged team members who are part of a positive culture are more likely to successfully implement the strategic plan put forth by practice leaders.

Strategic planning takes time and should be done at least once a year. It's best to devote one or more days to hold planning sessions outside the practice. Some practices schedule an annual weekend retreat to do strategic planning. You may want to consider hiring an outside facilitator or consultant with strategic planning experience to guide the leadership team if the budget allows for this expenditure. Facilitators are particularly helpful for large practices that have multiple owners and managers.

There are some pitfalls to be aware of when engaging in strategic planning. The last thing you want is to waste time on developing plans that never get implemented or to feel like the whole process was just an exercise on paper. Here are best practices that will help you avoid that scenario.

- Think about why you are engaging in strategic planning. Is it because you need to develop your vision or core values? Are you concerned about staying competitive? Do you simply want to establish goals for the year? Answering these types of questions ensures you have an appropriate agenda and clearly defined, desirable outcome for the process.
- Decide who to include in your strategic planning sessions. Who are the key stakeholders and employees that need to attend? The entire leadership team should be present and it's also helpful to include the team in at least part of the process. By involving all interested parties, you capture more ideas, solicit valuable

feedback, ensure there is consensus for decisions, and gain better buy-in from the team on action steps needed to implement strategic plans.

- For strategic planning to be effective, clearly define follow-up action steps as well as a timeline.
- Schedule time throughout the year for the leadership team to evaluate progress on implementing the practice's strategic plan. Track monthly or quarterly progress towards achieving goals outlined in the plan.

Developing Mission and Vision

The mission can be thought of as the purpose of a business or why it exists. Sometimes mission and vision statements are used interchangeably when referring to the medium to long term goals of the company.[2] However, most businesses differentiate the vision as a lofty or inspirational statement that creates a picture of what the company would look like upon achieving all goals.[3] Here is an excellent example of how the Mayo Clinic Health System differentiates their mission and vision:

The Mayo Clinic mission is "To inspire hope, and contribute to health and well-being by providing the best care to every patient through integrated clinical practice, education and research."

Their vision is "Mayo Clinic will provide an unparalleled experience as the most trusted partner for health care."[4]

The mission and vision relate closely to culture because the team is responsible for helping the company achieve its mission and vision. When everyone understands and believes in the mission and vision, they are more connected to the business and more invested in their work. Therefore, the leadership team must bring to life the mission and vision, or the statements are just meaningless words on paper. To maintain the visibility of the mission and vision, consistently remind employees of the valuable work they do to fulfill the purpose of the practice. Even though team members know their job duties, it's easy on a busy day to forget the "why" of providing quality care. Let everyone know that all their actions help preserve the human-animal bond. Likewise, if the vision of the practice is for "pet owners to feel like they're a member of our family as a result of our outstanding patient and client care", you can routinely convey how every client interaction helps the practice achieve this vision.

If you don't already have a mission and vision, you can develop these statements during the strategic planning process. Brainstorm answers to the following questions to draft an initial mission statement.

- Why do we exist?
- What is our purpose?
- Why do we do what we do?
- What is our business about?
- How do we fit into the community?
- What is important about our business?

Here are questions to answer to draft an initial vision statement.

- What are our medium to long-term goals?
- What is our most lofty goal?
- What feelings do we want to evoke for our clients?
- What is the greatest, highest purpose of our practice?
- What would it look like if we were the best veterinary hospital?
- What would it look like for our clients and patients if we achieved all our goals?

To capture the best ideas and feedback, distribute these questions to all participants of the strategic planning session prior to the meeting. Then facilitate a discussion to distill the preferred words and phrases from the answers into statements for consideration.

If your practice already has a written mission and vision, review the statements to see if they accurately reflect the current status of the practice. If they were drafted many years prior, the leadership team and other aspects of the business may have changed, or they may just need a refresh to be more relevant or succinct.

Swot Analysis

A SWOT analysis is a process used to evaluate business performance and the best strategies to maintain or improve the competitive position or profitability of the company. SWOT stands for strengths, weaknesses, opportunities, and threats. The evaluation of strengths and weaknesses is an internal assessment of what the business is doing well and where improvement is needed.

For example, strengths of a veterinary practice might be having a great location, high quality equipment, excellent doctors, and long-term employees. The same practice might have weaknesses related to breakdowns in internal communication, low client compliance rates, and ineffective team training programs.

With respect to strengths, consider if it creates a competitive advantage for the company. The practice may have excellent doctors but maybe all the surrounding practice do as well. However, if a doctor has advanced skills in ultrasonography or dentistry as well as outstanding client communication skills, this can be a competitive advantage that helps to attract pet owners, increase compliance, and increase client referrals.

The analysis of opportunities and threats is an external assessment to identify how the business can improve and factors that might influence the success of the company. Weaknesses of the practice can create opportunities. For the practice with low rates of compliance, there is an opportunity to implement strategies to improve client compliance which would in turn increase revenues and enhance profitability. In terms of threats, the practice may have risks associated with a shortage of doctors, negative hospital reviews, competition from other area providers, and weather damage to the building. When considering threats, think about both current and possible future threats. (See Figure 2.1 for an example veterinary practice SWOT Analysis.)

Figure 2.1 Example Veterinary Practice SWOT Analysis

	Strengths:	**Weaknesses:**
Internal environment	• CVTs with advanced expertise • High quality equipment • Attractive hospital • Excellent reputation • Friendly, caring team	• Lack of training for new hires • Breakdowns in internal communications • Inefficiency and excessive client wait times • Missed charges
External environment	**Opportunities:** • Implement new hire training program and protocol to capture missed charges • Expand capacity • Increase dental compliance • Leverage use of technology to improve team and client communications	**Threats:** • Loss of key employees • Decrease in client retention • Economic downturn • New competitors • Poor reviews online

The SWOT analysis is typically completed annually as part of strategic planning. Ideally, the entire team should participate so leadership teams can gather as much information as possible about what's working well and what's not working well. Sometimes team members have different knowledge and perspectives that you might not be aware of. For example, they may report breakdowns in internal communication as a factor related to low compliance rates. This is invaluable information since strategies to increase client compliance aren't likely to be as effective as desired without addressing how to improve communication between team members.

When doing a SWOT analysis, focus on brainstorming ideas and thoughts not on problem-solving. This doesn't mean you don't fully explore team input. It's helpful to ask questions and flesh out details related to any feedback. But if the team gets too caught up in debating topics, you may inadvertently shut down the creative process. In addition, be mindful of how much weight to give to specific discussion points. Is an issue agreed upon by most of the team or just a complaint of one employee? Encourage everyone to provide information and it is the job of practice leaders to assess the relative value of it when setting business goals.

Setting Business Goals

To avoid the pitfall of having a SWOT analysis that is just multiple lists on paper, be sure to use the evaluation to establish goals for the business. What did you learn from the SWOT analysis?

It makes sense to set goals to keep doing what is working well. If previous strategies to increase dental compliance were effective, for example, then set new goals to continue these tactics. On the other hand, if you determine a need to attract new clients and current initiatives aren't successful, then it's time to try new strategies.

Strive to organize and prioritize the SWOT information. To do this, decide on the most important ideas and action steps for each category. Identify your top three strengths, weaknesses, opportunities, and threats. Then develop goals related to these first. Once goals are set, solicit the team's ideas and feedback on how to best achieve the goals. This helps to gain their buy-in and consensus for the strategies they'll be responsible for implementing. In addition, encourage team members to offer regular feedback on their progress towards reaching goals.

Practice owners and managers tend to primarily think about setting marketing goals for the business when doing a SWOT analysis. In Chapter 10 on Marketing and Client Communications, you will read more about setting SMART goals to best market the practice. But the SWOT analysis is also a useful tool to identify goals related to operations, team development and human resource management. Through the strategic planning process, you may recognize the need to establish goals to improve operational efficiency, enhance training programs, or implement strategies to increase employee engagement.

ESTABLISHING CORE VALUES

Defining and establishing written core values for your business is an essential part of strategic planning. Recall from the last chapter, you discovered that providing clarity regarding the practice's mission, vision and core values was one of the characteristics of trusted leaders. Without defined core values, you may not be successful in developing the culture you want.

What Is a Core Value?

Core values are the beliefs, principles, commitments, ideals, philosophies, or standards that are most important to a company. They are set forth by the business owner(s) and leadership team. Core values are words or statements that define *how* a company will conduct business. For veterinary practices, the core values encompass the set of values with respect to how everyone in the business will interact with each other, patients, clients, and the community. Core values are generally listed on the company website and may be included on marketing collateral such as brochures, business cards, and social media platforms. The core values should also be included in the employee handbook. (See text box, "List of core values".)

To clearly convey the meaning of a core value, ideally each word or phrase should include a brief description that communicates how the core value will be upheld. For example, one of the core values for Southwest Airlines is "Wow our Customers." That can mean something different to different people. Southwest describes the core value this way: "Deliver world-class Hospitality. Create memorable connections. Be famous for friendly service."[5] Whether you like flying Southwest airlines or not, they do have a reputation for living this core value. Employees are generally friendly, welcoming, and known for having fun with customers. An example of a different approach is the Mayo Clinic Health System which states their core values in one statement as "The needs of the patient come first."[6] Their value-based philosophy is for everyone in the organization to always focus on patient needs when doing their job. Here is an example of a descriptor for a veterinary practice with a core value of compassion:

Compassion: We will treat all our patients and clients with kindness and respect. We strive to make sure every pet and client feels safe and comfortable.

If your practice doesn't have written core values, then be sure to devote time to creating them as they are a critical part of any business. Core values support all business activities and employee communications as you will see in the following chapters. Most businesses have four to ten core values. There isn't a magic number but if you have less than four, consider whether you've captured all the values that are meaningful for the business. Likewise, if you have more than ten, think about whether it feels like they are

LIST OF CORE VALUES

- High quality care
- Patients first
- Compassion
- Kindness
- Empathy
- Respect
- Integrity
- Communication
- Teamwork
- Accountability
- Innovation
- Continuous learning
- Knowledge
- Dedication
- Loyalty
- Excellence
- Understanding
- Passion
- Professionalism
- Service
- Creativity
- Honesty
- Trust
- Caring
- Discovery
- Responsibility
- Patient advocacy
- Authenticity
- Commitment
- Competence
- Cooperation
- Collaboration
- Diversity
- Fairness
- Gratitude
- Growth
- Well-being
- Progressive medical care
- Initiative
- Patience
- Inclusion
- Humility
- Consistency
- Servant leadership
- Dependability
- Courage
- Do the right thing

just a list. Perhaps some are essentially the same. For example, rather than having both integrity and honesty as core values, you could choose one and use the other word in the description.

If your practice already has core values, carefully evaluate them, and answer these questions:

- Are they still relevant?
- Do you have clear descriptions for each core value?
- Do they represent what is most important to the current owners and stakeholders?
- Has the business changed since they were drafted?
- Do you need to add or modify any of the values?
- Do your values sound like a slogan or tagline instead of expressing real values?

Helping Teams Understand Your Core Values

Sometimes core values are established without input from team members. This occurs when owners develop core values before starting their business. It may happen when businesses undergo a merger or acquisition. If a business is experiencing problems and needs strong leadership, it may roll out new core values. Otherwise, it's best to include the entire team in planning sessions on developing core values. Team members included in the strategic planning process have a better understanding of the core values. They gain greater appreciation for why they're important and are more likely to buy-in to future discussions about how their behavior must align with the core values. (See Figure 2.2 for a worksheet to use to ask the team for their input on developing core values.)

To ensure your culture is based on everyone living the core values, engage team members in dialogue about what behaviors align with the values and which ones violate them. Ideally, you would involve the team in this conversation when you first develop the practice's core values. But the discussion about how to live the practice's core values can occur at any time and in fact should be on-going. Let's say, for example, your practice has a core value of teamwork. Your team might identify the following work-related behaviors during a team meeting.

Behaviors that support our core value of Teamwork:

- Be willing to stay late to help others finish their job duties
- Say "Yes, I can help you" when co-workers ask for assistance

- Problem-solve together on the best way to accomplish goals
- Ask fellow co-workers "How can I help" when you see they are struggling

Behaviors that violate our core value of Teamwork:

- Never willing to cover shifts for others when they need time off
- Showing up late for work
- Only focusing on finishing your work rather than being willing to help teammates
- Saying "No, I can't help you, find someone else."

Figure 2.2: Team Worksheet for Developing Core Values

TEAM WORKSHEET FOR DEVELOPING CORE VALUES

The leadership team is in the process of defining our core values and would like your feedback.

Description of Core Values

Core values are words or statements that define how a company will conduct business. Companies may refer to their core values as "our beliefs", "our promise", "our commitments", "our principles" or "standards". A core value can be one word or a phrase. Our core values will encompass those values that define how all team members of the practice will interact with each other, pets, clients and the community.

Your Assignment

Please submit 3-5 core values for consideration. This is a brainstorming exercise so feel free to submit one word, a phrase and/or examples of what we do that represents our core values.

Your participation is greatly appreciated. Everyone's feedback will be collated and help us draft our final core values.

The deadline for this assignment: _____

Figure 2.3: Strategic Planning Worksheet

STRATEGIC PLANNING WORKSHEET

Strategic planning involves developing the practice's mission, vision, core values and business strategy. It also includes a SWOT Analysis and defining short & long-term practice goals.

Mission

The mission refers to your daily purpose. It encompasses who you serve, what need you satisfy and how you are serving these needs. A mission statement is often used in marketing collateral and doesn't change frequently.

What is the primary mission of your business? Brainstorm aspects of your purpose and then draft a one to two sentence mission statement.

_____

_____

Vision

The vision statement is an inspiring, motivating statement that refers to your long-term aspirations and goals. Think of creating a picture for the entire team-what you want to anchor them to. Your vision may be a lofty expression of your goal or simple statement about what the business wants to achieve.

What are medium to long-term goals of the owners/organization? What is your most lofty goal?

Brainstorm key points of your vision and then draft a one to two sentence statement.

_____

_____

Goals

What are your primary goals or objectives? (Consider both short and long-term goals.)

_____

_____

Figure 2.3: Strategic Planning Worksheet (continued)

Core values

Core values are guiding standards, beliefs, commitments, or principles. They reference "how" you will do business and speak to your practice culture.

What core values represent what is most important to you, your employees, and your clients? What core values drive how you will act and how you want everyone in the practice to act?

_____

_____

SWOT analysis

Internal Assessment

Strengths: What does your practice do really well? What about your practice helps you to be successful?

_____

_____

Weaknesses: What does your practice have difficulty with? What are areas needing improvement?

_____

_____

External Assessment

Opportunities: What could you do that would improve your competitive position in the marketplace? What could you do to turn your weaknesses into opportunities?

_____

_____

Threats: What could threaten your success?

_____

_____

MAKING YOUR DESIRED CULTURE A REALITY

Now that you know the value of strategic planning, how it relates to enhancing practice culture, and have thought about what type of culture you want, the next step is to recognize key management activities that will help you get where you want to go.

Create a Values-Based Culture

Having a values-based organization or values-based culture means everyone in the business shares and acts in accordance with the same core values. It means owners, leaders, and employees all live the values of the company.[7] It can take a significant amount of time to develop a values-based culture. One of the best examples of a values-based organization is Zappos. The former CEO of Zappos, Tony Hsieh, explained how the company gradually grew into a hugely profitable business that was acquired by Amazon by focusing on culture and core values. In his book, *Delivering Happiness*, he illuminated how the number one priority at Zappos is the culture and how they wanted their ten core values "to be reflected in everything we do."[8]

In a values-based culture, managers use the core values to guide actions and decisions; this can be thought of as managing by core values. This approach involves connecting all areas of management and team communications to the core values. The business's core values are the foundation for management; they are guiding principles for owners, managers, and the team. Discussions about core values become a part of recruitment, employee engagement strategies, team training, accountability meetings, performance evaluations, conflict resolution sessions, operational decisions, and leadership decisions. Examples of how to use core values in team communications will be presented in chapters 3-7.

Professionalism

Veterinarians graduate with a degree that carries with it a significant measure of credibility, status, and respect. They are now veterinary professionals which simply means they are affiliated with a specific profession. The term professional implies that someone has training, education, credentials, certification, or expertise and that they have met standards for their profession. The Merriam-Webster dictionary defines professionalism as "the conduct, aims, or qualities that characterize or mark a profession or a professional person."[9] But what exactly are those qualities? What is the conduct of a professional? Do you have to have a degree to act with professionalism?

Managers and practice owners who want to build a positive culture should encourage and demand professionalism from everyone on the team, not just the veterinarians. Professionalism is about following a code of conduct that upholds the standards of the profession. This means team members need to adhere to all medical standards, be committed to delivering high quality care, act with integrity, and never lose sight of the trust that has been granted by pet owners. Another way to think about professionalism is that it is acting in accordance with the core values of the practice.

To make professionalism part of the culture, begin by drafting a written code of conduct or professionalism policy statement. Unquestionably, this document should reference the practice core values but may further describe the need to demonstrate collegiality, maintain confidentiality, treat everyone with respect, and treat all patients and clients with dignity. As with the core values of the business, regularly engage team members in a discussion about behaviors that either uphold or violate the code of conduct. Otherwise, your professional code of conduct might become meaningless words on paper.

Encouraging Teamwork

In her book, *Making the Team: A Guide for Managers*, Leigh Thompson explains the difference between a team and a working group. Team members share a common goal and cannot achieve their objectives without helping each other. People in working groups share ideas and help each other but they work toward individual goals.[10] This is a relevant distinction because sometimes employees become so focused on their own job duties that they lose sight of the common goals of the business.

To encourage teamwork, look for evidence that the practice has one or more working groups instead of a team. Here are two examples that come to mind. Perhaps you observe that one of your client service representatives (CSRs) doesn't answer phones as often as her co-workers. You may see she stays in the back office to complete her administrative job duties even when there is a line of clients at the front desk. Likewise, you may notice an assistant who made a client wait ten minutes before admitting their pet to the hospital because they chose to first finish unpacking some inventory items.

Even though managers strive to build a culture that fosters teamwork, problems arise if team members don't know (or don't focus on) their common goals. To promote teamwork, make sure everyone understands that being part of a team means working together to complete daily work. Looking at the above examples, team members may need clarity about their job expectations, roles, and priorities. You would want to convey to both employees the need to immediately help their busy co-workers and assist clients rather than focusing on non-urgent job duties. You might also assign specific job roles to team members so it's clear how they can best work together to serve clients.

Recognize too, that the team's primary overarching common goal is set forth in the practice's mission and vision. Even in a sophisticated, service industry like veterinary medicine, it's easy for employees to become task-oriented and only focus on the next job duty without seeing the big picture. Busy veterinary teams may lose sight of the company WHY and the value of engaging in specific activities to help pets and people. Team members help to fulfill the mission and vision by working in partnership to achieve the hospital's goals. Let's say your practice has a quarterly goal to increase client compliance for medical progress exams. To increase appointment bookings, the entire team needs to be involved. The veterinarian needs to make appropriate recommendations based on the hospital's standards. A technician or assistant should communicate the value of the follow-up exam when reviewing take-home instructions with the client. And whoever checks the pet owner out should forward book the next appointment. If one team member doesn't do their part, the common goal to increase client compliance may not be met.

In his book, *The Five Dysfunctions of a Team*, Patrick Lencioni writes about common difficulties organizations face when attempting to achieve teamwork. His model to improve teamwork focuses on building trust, encouraging healthy conflict, gaining team commitment, increasing accountability, and making sure the team works to achieve the results and rewards of a common goal.[11] Managers can use the team assessment in the book to gauge how well they're doing in promoting teamwork.

PROMOTING DIVERSITY, EQUITY, AND INCLUSION

The company employee handbook needs to include a nondiscrimination/anti-harassment policy which clearly states the employer prohibits discrimination on the basis of gender, race, color, religion, national origin, age, disability status, sex, sexual orientation, gender identity, and marital status as well as statements that any form of harassment will not be tolerated. These policies exist to outline unacceptable behaviors, safeguard the rights of employees, and demonstrate the business complies with all federal, state, and local laws. (You will find more information on legal issues and avoiding discrimination in Chapter 5.)

The diversity, equity, and inclusion (DE&I) policy is uniquely different from the nondiscrimination/anti-harassment policy because it represents the desired culture of a business. While a business may not have any unlawful discriminatory or harassment practices, it may not actively promote diversity, equity, and inclusion. A DE&I policy should also be included in the employee handbook clearly stating the company's commitment to fostering a culture that promotes and celebrates the diversity of all team members. An example of a diversity policy can be found on the Society of Human Resource Management website.[12]

Of course, a policy statement isn't enough to promote a culture of diversity and inclusion. To do this, start by understanding (and helping your team understand) what diversity, equity and inclusion means and how it would look in your veterinary practice. Diversity in the workplace refers to team members that are different based on demographics such as age, race, religion, sexual orientation, gender, and socio-economic status. Diversity is also related to personality styles, family of origin, education level, and social or political views.

A commitment to diversity doesn't necessarily mean a company supports equity and is inclusive. Equity is the fair treatment of everyone in the company and ensuring that all employees have access to the same opportunities. Inclusion at work is about welcoming everyone and making sure they have a sense of belonging.[13] Not only does a practice that promotes diversity and inclusion strive to hire and retain a diverse group of employees, it also implements strategies and training to make sure all team members feel included (See textbox, "Promoting Inclusion in the Workplace").

The need to promote diversity and inclusion in the veterinary profession is clear. The U.S. Census statistics for 2019 show the profession is largely White (Non-Hispanic) with 89.1% of veterinarians being White.[14] Charlotte Hansen, assistant director of statistical analysis for the AVMA, reported at the 2020 AVMA Economic Summit that 92% of the profession is White, 4% is Hispanic/Latino, 3% is Asian and 1% is Black. (See Figure 2.4: Race and Ethnicity in Veterinary Medicine.) In recent years, multiple national organizations have increased their efforts to improve awareness about the lack of diversity in veterinary medicine. Associations that actively promote diversity and inclusion in the profession include AVMA, AAHA, the National Association for Black Veterinarians, Association of American Veterinary Medical Colleges (AAVMC), Multicultural Veterinary Medical Association (MCVMA) and PrideVMC which has a mission to "create a better world for the LGBTQ+ veterinary community."[15]

Enhancing the Hospital Culture

PROMOTING INCLUSION IN THE WORKPLACE:

- Actively seek the ideas and feedback of all team members during team meetings to make sure everyone's voice is heard.

- Ensure all projects are inclusive. Managers can ask themselves: Does this project include diverse members? Are all views being heard? Who hasn't yet been involved with a project?

- Acknowledge holidays for all cultures and adjust policies to allow time off for floating holidays.

- Facilitate team meetings and provide education on DE&I at least annually.

- Have potluck lunches or bring in food to celebrate different cultures.

- Recognize and celebrate various groups and important months such as Black History month in February and LGBT Pride month in June.

Figure 2.4: Race and Ethnicity in Veterinary Medicine

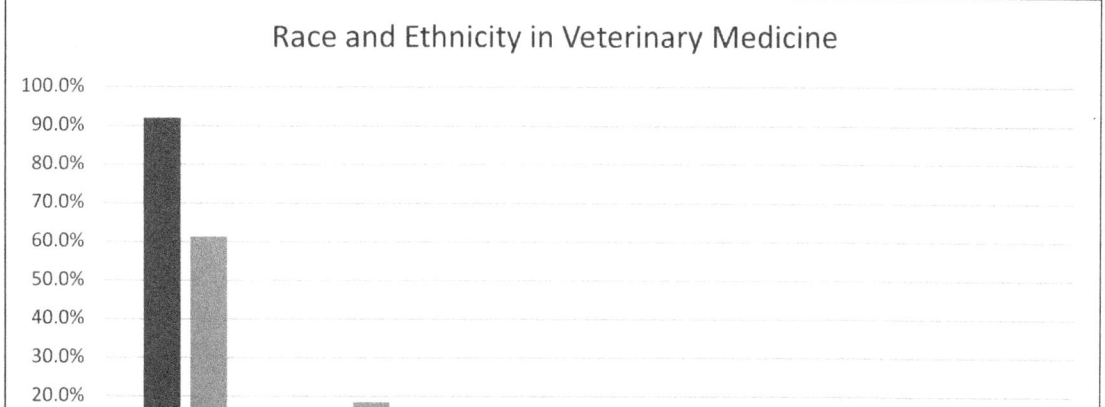

Source: 2019 AVMA and U.S. Census Data

There are many benefits to promoting diversity and inclusion in the workplace. Perhaps the most obvious one is increasing the ability of the organization to attract and retain the most talented employees. Remember that the millennial generation (25-40 years old in 2021) is the most diverse generation to date, and Generation Z (born after 1997) is even more diverse. It is worth noting that millennials, who will make up 75% of the workforce by 2025, actively seek to work for companies that promote diversity and making sure everyone's voice is heard.[16] Another major benefit of having a culture that embraces diversity, equity and inclusion is that it supports well-being for the team; employees have a greater sense of belonging and experience higher levels of trust in the company's leadership. Having a diverse and inclusive culture has been proven to increase creativity, employee engagement and productivity.

Overcoming Unconscious Bias

Part of diversity and inclusion training includes helping teams understand and know how to eliminate unconscious bias. Vanderbilt University defines unconscious bias as "prejudice or unsupported judgments in favor of or against one thing, person, or group as compared to another, in a way that is usually considered unfair." As with discrimination, unconscious bias tends to be exhibited towards people based on their minority status related to race, ethnicity, sexual orientation, religion, gender, age, or disability just to name a few.[17] Unconscious bias is a result of learned stereotypes and attitudes that result in behaviors towards other people or treatment of others that is either preferential or unfavorable.

Unconscious bias, which is also termed implicit bias, takes many forms. One that is more commonly known is the horns or halo effect which means we view a person either positively or unfairly based on a characteristic.[18] For example, if a veterinarian graduated from one of the top five veterinary schools in the United States, they may be viewed as being smart and talented. Likewise, if someone is tall and well-dressed, they are frequently viewed as being competent and responsible (the halo effect). An example of the horns effect takes place when an employee is viewed as being less knowledgeable or skilled on the basis of a perceived negative characteristic such as their accent, weight, voice tone or attire. Here are a few other examples of unconscious bias.

- Name bias occurs when people are judged based on their name during the hiring process. Studies have found people with African American or Asian names on their resumes receive fewer call backs.[19]

- Assuming a job candidate or employee with children won't be willing to switch shifts.
- Thinking an older employee isn't tech savvy and won't be adept with the practice software program.
- Making job assignments based on gender or ethnicity. For example, assuming that a Latino employee won't be good working at the front desk because they are too loud or that a male employee is best suited to be a team leader.
- Matching mentors and mentees based on gender, race, and age.

Managers can take the following action steps to help eliminate unconscious bias in the workplace.

- Ensure the leadership team commits to increasing their knowledge about unconscious bias and how to adopt behaviors and policies that promote diversity and inclusion.
- Make sure the vision, mission and core values of the practice reflect a commitment to diversity and inclusion.
- Provide relevant team training in the form of seminars, reading material, and workshops.
- Facilitate team discussions at least a few times a year where employees have a safe space to discuss possible bias and ask for what they need.
- Use online assessment tools to identify actions the organization can take.
- Take the Implicit Association Test (IAT), an online assessment at the Project Implicit website (https://implicit.harvard.edu/implicit/).[20]

Committing to Anti-Racism

Historically, racism has been defined as being prejudiced against someone on the basis of their skin color. The word not only refers to the actions of an individual but also can refer to a society or organization. The author of the best-selling book *How to be an Antiracist*, Ibram X. Kendi, more broadly defines racism as all the race-based societal disparities and the need to oppose all systems that exist within ourselves and the world.[21]

One of the ways to create a culture free of racism is to identify and eliminate any form of micro-aggression in the workplace. Micro-aggression is defined by Merriam-Webster as "a comment or action that subtly and often unconsciously or unintentionally expresses a prejudiced attitude toward a member of a marginalized group (such as a racial minority)."[22] Micro-aggression includes making racist jokes, referencing stereotypes about a group, and giving preferential treatment to white employees. Sometimes, people make comments without thinking or realizing they are racist such as telling a black co-worker that they are "so articulate" or referring to a marginalized group as "you people."[23] (See text box, "Examples of racism and microaggressions in the workplace.")

When thinking about how to create and support a culture free of racism, it isn't enough to simply have a policy statement but rather managers need to be proactive to provide training and implement antiracist programs. A starting point is to complete an internal assessment of all employee policies and communications related to hiring, performance reviews, accountability meetings, and promotions to determine whether the business actively promotes being antiracist. Practices should also reflect on whether strategies exist to attract Latino/Hispanic and Black/African American pet owners, for example, as well as how the team treats non-white clients.

Another important action is to promote open communication and the ability for teams to have uncomfortable conversations. Lisa Greenhill, senior director for institutional research and diversity at AAVMC, writes about the need to avoid tone policing which is essentially shutting down or discounting conversations about controversial topics especially when someone becomes passionate, angry, or emotional when speaking. Tone policing might take the form of discounting remarks such as "I can't talk to you when you're being irrational" or "Just calm down and be an adult." Tone policing can be problematic because it shuts down dialogue, shared understanding, conflict-resolution, and problem-solving.[24]

Another concept to be aware of is performative allyship which is taking action such as condemning racism but not actually completing steps necessary to rid the organization of racism. Put another way, it is stating you care but not implementing measures to support marginalized groups.[25] To avoid the pitfall of simply paying lip service to being antiracist, think about actions you can take to achieve a specific outcome. This includes an evaluation of hiring procedures, calling out unacceptable behavior, implementing diversity training, and fostering a culture of inclusiveness.

Celebrating Employee Differences

A big part of promoting diversity and inclusion is to embrace and celebrate employee differences. One not discussed yet is that of generational differences. Practices may

> **EXAMPLES OF RACISM AND MICROAGGRESSIONS IN THE WORKPLACE**
>
> Aside from flagrant racial discrimination, there are many subtle forms of racism and multiple microaggressions that teams need to be made aware of. Here are examples:
>
> - Expressing concerns about a job applicant with an ethnic or foreign name
> - Not giving a person from an ethnic of minority group the same consideration as a white job candidate
> - Assumptions that someone from another country isn't as educated
> - Asking an individual who is black where they are from
> - Commenting to a U.S. born Hispanic/Latino person that they speak English well
> - Stating that someone must have gotten into a prestigious college or promoted because they're African American
> - Making jokes about an ethnic or racial group or their customs
> - Telling someone their name is so hard to pronounce
> - Making comments about a Black/African American woman's natural hair
> - Telling someone who is gay or transgender that they don't look like it
> - Avoiding sitting next to co-workers who are different based on their racial, ethnic, or sexual orientation
> - Saying comments such as "that's so gay" or "I jewed him down on the price."
> - Telling someone of Asian descent "You should be great at doing this" when referring to calculating a drug dose

have team members from four or even five different generations. People from different generations have unique perspectives, ideas, insight, skills, and lived experiences. Take care to avoid stereotypes or assumptions about the needs and wants of each generation. This means, for example, eliminating a stereotype that younger generations don't have as good a work ethic as older generations or assumptions that older employees aren't tech savvy.

Interestingly, a study looking at the value baby boomers, Generation X, and Generation Y (millennials) place on various workplace characteristics associated with "best places to work" found that there were more similarities than differences for the

3 generations. For example, all groups valued work-life balance and training opportunities. Although the differences weren't that large, millennials did place more value on career advancement opportunities, diversity climate, and immediate recognition and feedback than older generations.[26] This study highlights the benefit of understanding generational differences but also how important it is to look at similarities as well rather than making assumptions based on an employee's age.

Cultures that promote diversity and inclusion ensure everyone is heard and respected regardless of their age, race, ethnicity, sexual orientation, religion, disability, or any other characteristic. As a manager, be sure to leverage the talent and strengths of everyone in the organization. Strive to create an atmosphere that honors the value that each employee brings to the practice. Actively seek the perspectives of all team members and encourage shared decision-making. Remember diversity leads to more ideas and better decisions. A business that celebrates diversity, not only creates a culture of respect and appreciation but it also fosters an environment that is supportive, welcoming, and even has a sense of family.

WORK-LIFE BALANCE AND WELL-BEING

Without some semblance of work-life balance and personal well-being, people eventually suffer from commonly known negative health effects such as fatigue, increased risk of cardiovascular disease, anxiety, and depression. Moreover, there are adverse effects on culture including a decrease in employee engagement, morale, and productivity.

Work-Life Strategies for Managers

Work-life balance refers to balancing the demands of the job with one's personal life and self-care. Some people have no problem with work-life balance while others with hectic jobs struggle to make time for themselves and/or their family. Work-life balance can be particularly difficult for parents and those who are caregivers for elderly, disabled or sick family members.

Veterinary practice owners and managers sometimes fall victim to thinking they should devote an unreasonable amount of time and energy to the business. This dedication can have a negative effect on the practice culture and personal relationships as a result of the associated stress and burn-out.

The first step to creating work-life balance is to assess what's working well and what's not working well. Are you working 40 hours a week, or do you average 55-60 hours per week? Do you work five days a week or more? Do you routinely give up time with family to do work on the weekend or at night? Are you always available to answer calls from employees after hours? What does your family think about how hard you work? Have you missed important events with family or friends? How long has it been since you had a vacation free of work? Understandably, there are times when practice managers must put in extra hours to handle a crisis but if this is a weekly occurrence, it suggests your work-life balance isn't working well.

Different work-life balance strategies work for different people and you may find you have to try multiple ones to see what works for you. Here are some proven ways to create better work-life balance.

- First, think about what is missing in your life or what feels out of balance. Is it that you don't have time with your family or friends? Do you lack time for exercise? Have hobbies and enjoyable activities been sidelined? What do you want to have more of in your life? Exploring answers to these questions can help you decide on plans to improve work-life balance.
- Create and commit to a schedule with blocks for personal time. Time blocks may be for days off for a vacation or for short periods of time away from work. For example, you may block off time to get out of the hospital for lunch (even if that isn't everyday), go to the gym, leave early for a family function, or to have one afternoon off each month.
- Increase your productivity (For more information, see Chapter 1 on Becoming a Successful Manager.)
- Set boundaries with team members. The reasons employees may call you after hours are rarely urgent. If you routinely take calls or texts after work, this in an indication you need better boundaries with your employees. To set boundaries, establish guidelines and expectations for the team regarding when it is acceptable to contact you after hours. You can also look for opportunities to empower employees. (To learn more about employee empowerment, see Chapter 6 on Employee Retention.)
- Commit to your health and fitness. Exercise regularly and avoid consuming too much junk food, sugar, and mid-day caffeine while at work.

In recent years, there has been talk about the concept of work-life integration leading people to ask if they may sometimes work from home. With work-life integration, work and personal time are not completely separate. Someone might engage in various activities at different times throughout the day. This type of schedule may work in some instances and the COVID-19 pandemic that started in 2020 showed how employees can be effective while working virtually. However, in most instances, veterinary managers will want to spend the majority of their time at the practice because of the need to interact one-on-one with practice leaders, team members and clients. One of the drawbacks of adopting a work-life integration schedule is that it could increase stress for managers because the lines between work and personal life blur. A different approach might be for managers to look at opportunities to increase the flexibility of their workday when needed.

Promoting a Culture of Work-Life Balance

Even when practice leaders recognize team members are overworked, they may justify the situation due to the demands of the business especially if they're stressed themselves. And team members often willingly take on extra hours and job stresses because they're dedicated to the practice. Employees may feel they have to accept extra hours because their work is so important, and they may even embrace being overworked like it is a badge of honor. As stated previously, this ultimately has negative effects on the hospital culture. In addition to improving their own work-life balance, practice owners and managers should seek to foster a culture that encourages work-life balance for the team as this leads to improved employee recruitment, job satisfaction, retention, and productivity.

Take care to monitor the amount of responsibility each employee has, the number of hours worked each week, and the type of hours worked. Unless a team member has a regular schedule to work Saturday and Sunday (E.g., employees who work at an 24/7 hospital, emergency practice or as a kennel attendant), it probably isn't healthy for them to work too many weekend hours. Likewise, consistent overtime suggests an employee doesn't have good work-life balance. And finally, if an employee is routinely receiving phone calls from co-workers after hours because of their area of responsibility, managers may want to intervene to establish appropriate boundaries with the team.

To promote a culture of work-life balance, try to eliminate (or at least minimize) overtime hours, insist employees take their vacation time, and avoid rewarding work warriors. People who work a high number of hours need to be acknowledged and appreciated but this shouldn't be seen as the only way to win favor and get ahead at the practice. Here are some long-term strategies to implement that support work-life balance.

- Embrace job sharing and/or the use of part-time employees to fill work shifts.
- Talk to each team member about their work-life balance. Ask what they need or desire and offer to help them implement a plan to reach their goals.
- Make sure employees take their meal and rest break.
- Ensure team members take their vacation or paid time off to rest and recharge.
- Consider perks, rewards or benefits related to better work-life balance such as health club memberships, a monthly subscription to a meal delivery service, gift cards for a restaurant or cleaning service, etc.
- Be willing to make schedule adjustments when the practice is short-staffed.

Enhancing Team Well-Being

Problems with stress, burn-out, compassion fatigue, and suicide have long been identified in the veterinary profession. The proportionate mortality rate (PMR) for suicide for U.S. veterinarians is higher than for the general population.[27] In addition to dealing with mortality and morbidity, today's veterinary teams experience even higher levels of stress and compassion fatigue due to the increasing demands of the job. This includes delivering more sophisticated patient care, responding to high expectations and demands of pet owners, and the shortage of credentialed veterinary technicians and doctors.

Practices should put in place programs that promote team well-being as well as work-life balance. Managers can take advantage of available resources from national organizations such as AVMA and AAHA. AVMA has webinars, a well-being certificate program, a stress test, stress and well-being survey, and multiple assessments on well-being. AAHA has several publications on practice team well-being and initiatives on how to have a healthy workplace culture. These tools and resources can be used to help implement well-being initiatives as well as a framework to create dialog with teams. Having open communication about physical and mental well-being helps to foster a culture that values health and wellness.

Given that team members spend many hours at work, look for ways to create an environment that is inviting and as stress-free as possible. Making changes to the break room, offices, and rest rooms is one way to do this. Ideas include adding plants, a massage chair, a yoga mat, and artwork that is visually calming or inspirational. Additionally, team members appreciate having comfortable outdoor seating to use when the weather is nice. Some practices have added games such as cornhole to their outdoor areas and interactive games such as Jenga in break rooms.

Managers do need to recognize that while they can lend an empathetic ear and promote well-being, they aren't therapists or trained counselors. Team members may need professional help and should be encouraged to seek outside assistance as appropriate. One resource is to have an employee assistance program (EAP) as a benefit for employees. These plans provide free, confidential resources such as counseling, personal assessments, and referrals to other services as needed. An EAP is a valuable employee benefit that all practices should consider offering.

SUMMARY

Your practice culture for better or worse has developed and may have changed over time. Reviewing the history of a practice often explains why and how the culture evolved to the present state. Cultures can be impacted by changes in ownership, leadership, team dynamics, policies or systems, the workplace environment, and outside societal influences. Regardless of the status of your current culture, you can affect positive change. Creating a desirable culture isn't really a destination so much as a process. You don't complete a set of actions that result in having a perfect culture but rather implement ongoing strategies that maintain and enhance the business culture. The foundation of this process is to engage in annual strategic planning including committing to a set of core values that will serve as a roadmap for all actions. Diversity, equity, inclusion, work-life balance, and a dedication to practice team well-being must all be incorporated in the core values, so they become embedded in the culture.

CHAPTER 3

Recruiting and Hiring Team Members

Recruitment has always been a challenge for veterinary practices given the need to hire employees who are uniquely qualified to provide medical care for animals and exceptional client care for pet owners. It's not easy to find team members who have the requisite skills sets to excel in veterinary medicine. To be successful, veterinary hospitals rely on talented veterinarians and technicians to utilize their advanced technical skills and client communication skills to generate revenue. Practices need team members who can deliver exceptional client service. In addition, most team members need to have some amount of training in the areas of veterinary terminology, preventive healthcare, and patient care.

Recruitment is also challenging because over the years, the profession has experienced a shortage of both credentialed veterinary technicians and veterinarians. During the 2019 AVMA Economic Summit, economists discussed the veterinarian shortage noting that unemployment of veterinarians in 2019 was only 0.8% and the number of searchable jobs on the AVMA Veterinary Career Center vastly exceeded the number of new job seekers. The demand for veterinarians (and paraprofessional staff) remained strong even during the COVID-19 pandemic that started in 2020. AVMA reported that the unemployment rate for veterinarian dropped to 0.7% and there was an increase in job postings compared to 2019. A 2016 survey by the National Association of Veterinary Technicians in America (NAVTA) identified low pay, compassion fatigue, burnout, and lack of recognition or career advancement as reasons behind the high turnover rate for technicians in clinical practice.

To address many of the challenges of credentialed technicians, NAVTA formed the Veterinary Nurse Initiative (VNI) in 2016. The VNI advocates changing the professional title of a credentialed veterinary technician to registered veterinary nurse to better inform pet owners about the work done by technicians. Their goals also include standardizing credentials in the U.S., promoting career advancement opportunities, and increasing recognition of the value and scope of credentialed technicians or nurses. Readers should be aware that this initiative has both supporters and critics. However, presumably everyone agrees that credentialed technicians should be fully empowered to use all their skills and promoting career opportunities can help with recruitment efforts.

All businesses need a clearly defined system for recruitment and hiring of employees. This is especially true for veterinary practices due to the difficulty in finding and retaining qualified team members. Always be on the lookout for talented team members. In fact, for many hospitals, recruitment has become an on-going activity. Having established protocols in place helps make the process more efficient. With advanced planning, managers can avoid feeling like they need to scramble to get ready every time a position is open. (See Table 3.2 for Recruitment Strategies Best Practices.)

DEFINING YOUR IDEAL CANDIDATE

One of the most overlooked aspects of recruitment is to define what type of employee the practice wants to hire. This helps ensure the hospital hires a team member that fits into the culture and effectively contributes to the practice rather than just hiring *someone* to fill a position. To define the desirable qualities in a new hire, first look at the core values of the business. As noted in the last chapter, core values serve as a roadmap for behavior at work; seek to hire people whose values align with those of the practice. In the section below on interviews, you will see examples of questions to ask candidates to assess their fit with your core values.

In addition, think about desired character traits, talents, and requisite skills for the job. Many jobs require hard skills which refers to the education, training, or technical skills a candidate must have or be able to acquire while on the job. Soft skills, on the other hand, refers to the personal qualities an employee must have to excel in their job and be a good fit for the culture. Job candidates for a client service representative position, for example, need to be proficient with computer software programs (hard skills) but they also need to enjoy talking to clients and have a talent for customer service (soft skills). Other examples of desirable traits for team members include reliability, a desire to learn, patience, staying calm under pressure and the ability to problem-solve. Recognize that these qualities and abilities aren't personality types but rather personal attributes. People with different types of personality can have the same preferred characteristics and talents.

In addition to identifying the desired values, abilities, and personal characteristics of the ideal candidate, define all other job requirements for a position prior to initiating the recruitment process. For example, most employees need to be able to lift 30 or more pounds. Another obvious job requirement is an employee's work schedule. Sometimes practices eager to find team members end up with employees who either can't or are unwilling to work the schedule or hours they were hired to fill. An example is hiring someone who doesn't want to work Saturdays or who can't stay till the hospital closes. These issues need to be worked out prior to hiring a job candidate to avoid problems related to work schedules, staffing and favoritism.

COMPENSATION AND BENEFITS

Recruitment can be highly competitive given that most practices are trying to find qualified team members. It doesn't help that pay wages have traditionally been low for most positions. Private practices in some locations may have the added difficulty of competing with corporate veterinary practices (or businesses in other industries) that have bigger payroll budgets. While compensation and benefits aren't the reason for people choosing veterinary medicine jobs, it's definitely a reason behind people leaving the profession or leaving for a better paying job at another hospital. Simply put, practices must pay competitive wages and offer benefits employees want to stay competitive.

Employers should ideally decide on pay ranges prior to engaging in recruitment for an open job position. Otherwise practice owners and managers are prone to make snap decisions and pay whatever it takes (or what they think is necessary) to secure a job candidate. This can result in two problems. First, team members who find out that a new employee with a similar position is making more than them easily become disgruntled. Second, employees may be brought on who are overpaid in relationship to the revenue they produce or their productivity.

To decide on compensation for each position, evaluate answers to these three questions.

1. What can the business afford? Staff and doctor payroll is one of the largest hospital expenses. The benchmark reported by AAHA for staff compensation as a percentage of gross revenues is an average of 18.9% for all hospitals. The 2019 Well Managed Practice (WMP) benchmarks reported staff compensation as a range of 22-25% of gross revenues. These benchmarks include the employees' portion of payroll taxes and WMP data includes retirement contributions. Be cautious of hiring employees at wages that would result in total staff compensation exceeding these amounts as it may affect the profitability of the practice. When hiring doctors, compensation can be tied to the amount of revenue produced which helps ensure the practice stays profitable. (See Chapter 9 for more information on Financial Management.)

2. What are competitive pay wages for the city or region? As a starting point, managers can look at national averages for veterinary staff wages. However, it's most important to take into consideration what wages need to be to stay competitive

in the area where the practice is located. Hourly wages for team members in major cities such as Los Angeles or New York are higher than in other parts of the U.S. Local competition may also affect wages. For example, if the practice is near corporate practices or specialty practices that offer higher wages, the business may have to pay higher wages to stay competitive. Of course, managers also need to pay attention to what the minimum wage is for their city and state.

3. What value or unique skills does the employee bring that may justify higher pay? Does the candidate have advanced training or skills, certifications, or talents? Examples include laser therapy certification, training in acupuncture, advanced surgical skills, advanced patient care skills, Fear Free certification, proficiency with software programs and possessing outstanding client communication skills.

Employee benefits can be an excellent recruitment tool if the practice offers benefits in line with what job candidates want. As with wages, it's essential to look at the benefits expense as a percentage of revenues to assess what the business can afford to pay. For most practices, employee benefits are 2-3% of revenues. In some instances, benefits are more valuable to an employee than wages, so managers need to consider both when deciding on the best way to attract team members. While it's the most costly for the business, health insurance is often the most desirable employee benefit. Practices that pay half or more of employee's monthly health insurance premium can likely attract more employees than those that don't provide this benefit. Offering dental, vision, life and disability insurance are all attractive benefits but may be cost prohibitive for smaller practices. Vacation and sick pay which are often offered together as paid time off (PTO) is particularly important to employees. The more time off, the better in the eyes of job candidates. And most employees appreciate the value of being able to contribute to a retirement account such as a 401K plan.

Other common benefits that help practices stay competitive include paying for uniforms, dues, licenses, and continuing education as well as offering health care discounts for employees' pets. In addition, consider offering less traditional benefits that would help recruit employees such as an employee assistance program (EAP), tuition reimbursement, gym memberships, wellness programs, flexible schedules, job-sharing, daycare for personal pets, child daycare, and profit-sharing bonuses.

Increasingly, practices have been offering to pay signing bonuses to veterinarians and credentialed veterinary technicians as a means to attract candidates. The AVMA reported that 30% of the respondents of their survey of 2019 graduates who accepted a private practice position received a signing bonus. If the practice pays say somewhere between $500 and $5,000, the money can help pay moving expenses and is enough to get the attention of job applicants. Paying a signing bonus is typically less expensive than hiring a recruiter and may well be worth the expense to secure a talented team member.

EFFECTIVE ADS

Once the need arises to hire a new employee, the next step is to advertise the job opening. The keys to successful advertising are knowing where to look for team members and how to write the best job ad for your open job position. (See Table 3.1: What to Include in Job Ads.)

Where To Place Ads

Since most people search the web when looking for a job, it makes sense to post ads almost exclusively on internet sites. In some instances, you may want to consider print ads as well. For example, print ads in veterinary journals are appropriate when conducting a nationwide search for an associate veterinarian. Likewise, print ads may be effective when placed in commonly read veterinary publications such as trade magazines or newsletters from state and local veterinary associations.

Managers may want to post job ads on multiple internet sites to maximize the chances of attracting the greatest number of qualified applicants. Identifying the best websites for job posts is based on knowing which sites job applicants routinely search and personal experience related to which sites seem to attract the most responses. Multiple national veterinary associations have career centers on their websites including AVMA, AAHA and VHMA. Another popular website used for recruitment is Indeed. Some managers have found success placing ads on their state veterinary medical association website, LinkedIn, and the company Facebook page.

In addition to posting job ads on websites, never underestimate the power of networking as a recruitment tool. It can be beneficial to interact with multiple colleagues to let them know about your job openings. Pharmaceutical or other company representatives that call on the practice can be a valuable means of getting the word out that you're hiring. They may know about employees who are unhappy in their current job or are looking to relocate to your area. It can also be beneficial to actively network with instructors at any veterinary technician college that is within a few hours distance from the practice.

Recruiters are another way to go for those practices that are struggling to find doctors, technicians, or a practice manager. Recruiters aren't inexpensive so it's advisable to talk to multiple companies to find out about their fees, process, and track record of success before hiring one.

Choose The Right Words

Strive to write a job ad that attracts the most applicants for your position. At a minimum, your ad should include the following:

- The job title for the position
- The name and city location of your hospital
- Any relevant job requirements
- A brief description of job duties
- Contact information and how to submit a resume.

Remember the goal is to recruit a pool of applicants with the right skills, talents and availability for your job opening. Be sure to include whether the job is full time or part time and relevant hours of the job such as the need to work Saturdays. One common mistake is failing to include job requirements such as the number of years of experience or requisite skills the job applicant must have to be considered for the position. If you're only interested in hiring a credentialed veterinary technician, for example, then make sure the job title includes the words "certification required" or "licensure preferred." Likewise, if you need a technician with advanced skills in anesthesia and surgery, then be sure to include this in your ad. If you want a receptionist with a talent for service, it's best to advertise for a "client service representative" to attract applicants with prior customer service experience.

Along with the brief description of job duties, it's advisable to include specific attributes about the type of employee you are recruiting. Your ad might state "we're looking for a self-motivated individual with a passion for patient care and client education." While this doesn't guarantee you'll attract the ideal candidate, it does let job applicants know relevant details about your position.

Another often overlooked aspect of an effective job ad is to include information which falls into the category of "what's in it for them." Since you're competing against other employers who actively seek team members, try to make your ad stand out. List any benefits you offer such as health insurance, a 401K, paid time off, paid holidays, uniform allowance, and continuing education. In addition, try to paint a picture of what it's like to work at your practice. Highlight benefits related to the work environment or location of the practice. This might include references to joining a friendly team, your commitment to diversity and inclusion, working in a beautiful state-of-the art facility, and opportunities for advancement. Including the practice's core values can also help attract employees.

Be sure to keep an electronic copy of all your job ads for each position in the practice so you'll always be ready for recruitment. Then you can simply review the ad before placement to make sure it accurately reflects details about your current job opening.

Table 3.1: What to Include in Job Ads

Information to Include	Example
Job title and job type	Client service representative (CSR), Full-time
Name and location of practice	ABC Veterinary Hospital, Nashville, TN
Job requirements and any qualifications	Must be available to work Saturdays Proficiency with MS Word Veterinary client service experience preferred
Ideal candidate description	We are searching for an outstanding, people-oriented candidate to join our team! Top applicants will have a positive, can-do attitude, excellent communication skills, and a passion for serving the needs of pet owners.
Description of job duties	Our CSRs handle phone calls, emails, text messages, and face-to-face communications with clients. Duties include accurate documentation in medical records, scheduling appointments, client education on basic preventive care, relaying information to doctors and other team members, and processing payments.
Compensation and Benefits	List pay range and major benefits
Non-monetary benefits	List any perks, opportunities, value of working at the practice, area activities
Contact information	Please submit cover letter and resume to manager@gmail.com List website

BECOMING A PREFERRED EMPLOYER

The report on Fortune's 100 Best Companies to Work for in 2019 revealed that 84% of employees at these companies look forward to coming to work and 83% said that management actions match their words. Specific reasons why employees wanted to work where they did was because of the company's "focus on values, trust, innovation, financial growth, leadership effectiveness, and maximizing the full human potential of every employee." Anyone looking for a job in industries represented by the top 100 companies would surely be attracted to these companies due to the positive reputation and the attributes of the culture.

While you may not be able to secure the kind of media press large companies enjoy, word of mouth in your local community and in the veterinary medicine community can definitely work in your favor. In fact, one of the top recruiting tools is to be known as a one of the best places to work in your community. It takes time to develop an outstanding reputation as a preferred employer. But having this long-term vision in mind is vital to recruitment efforts.

Building the Hospital Reputation

Both employer actions and those of employees can build or break down the company's reputation. Everyone on the team needs to understand the role they play in enhancing the hospital reputation and how their behavior reflects on the practice either positively or negatively. For example, if an employee wearing scrubs with the hospital logo acts rudely or says something unkind when outside the practice, this creates a negative impression of the business. Similarly, team members who eat lunch locally and are always friendly create positive impressions of the business.

Monitoring online reviews of the practice is a marketing activity but also important for recruitment. Job candidates will undoubtedly look online for information about the company and review the business website. If the practice has negative reviews, they may have concerns about working there. This is another reason it's essential to encourage positive reviews from clients and respond to negative reviews (See Online Reputation Management in Chapter 10.)

Of course, the best way to build the hospital reputation is to have a positive culture. When practices pay low wages, have limited benefits, high employee turnover, an unsafe work environment or toxic employees, people in the profession looking for jobs tend to find out this information. On the other, the same is true about having a great culture.

Current and past team members, veterinary sales representatives, clients, and area colleagues can all sing the praises of a practice they know is a wonderful place to work.

In the last chapter, you learned ways to enhance the hospital culture. Don't be afraid to actively seek out opportunities to promote your culture and the value of working at your practice. You can do this at networking events, when visiting area businesses, at community events, and on the practice website. The secret is to always promote the business even when you're not recruiting for a specific job position. Tell people why your practice is a great place to work and be as descriptive as possible. For example, in addition to mentioning competitive compensation, you might highlight positive aspects of the culture such as taking part in team-building activities, promoting work-life balance, having wellness programs, and being committed to diversity and inclusion.

Another way to build the hospital reputation is to implement a mentorship program. Mentors are team members with more experience than the mentee who is usually a new team member or someone with less experience. Mentors provide support, knowledge and expertise that helps mentees succeed in the workplace. AAHA has established guidelines for mentorship as well as a mentorship accreditation program. Usually, practices only think of mentorship programs for veterinarians who are new graduates. But mentorship programs can be implemented for all job roles and are an excellent way to help new employees successfully integrate into the practice. Likewise, mentorship programs can be used to help employees learn and grow professionally.

Increasing Awareness

Being active in the community is an excellent way to increase awareness for the business and attract job candidates., People appreciate working for companies committed to social responsibility. Younger generations often explore and seek out businesses that give back to the community. Veterinary practices can become involved with volunteer efforts or community events in many ways. This may include holding a blood drive at the hospital, collecting food and supplies for local animal shelters, helping the homeless, and educating school children about careers in veterinary medicine, just to name a few.

Bear in mind that only occasionally participating in community activities isn't likely to enhance the hospital's reputation enough to significantly affect recruitment. Instead, the practice must be known for its on-going efforts and commitments. The hospital might, for example, develop a positive reputation because every year the team schedules a few days to provide pet care to underserved communities or the entire hospital team does charitable work every few months.

Table 3.2: Recruitment Strategies Best Practices

Recruitment Strategies	Description
Define your ideal candidate	• Find team members with aligned core values • Identify desired skills, talents, and character traits • Confirm job requirements and needs of the practice • Decide on areas of flexibility, e.g., part-time vs. full-time, hours worked, schedule
Compensation and benefits	• Determine hospital budget and maximum wages the hospital can afford • Identify competitive compensation for your area • Draft a list of all benefits and associated value • Consider signing bonuses or other perks
Write effective job ads	• Identify the best online sites to post your position • Write attention grabbing ads that include relevant information as well as benefits • Highlight non-monetary benefits such as mentoring, reasons to live in your area and advantages of working at the business
Networking	• Talk to your vendors about open positions • Join community organizations • Use LinkedIn and social media sites to promote job openings
Build your hospital reputation as a preferred provider	• Promote your core values, community involvement, charitable activities, and opportunities for employee development on website and when networking • Become active in the community • Monitor your online reputation • Enhance team morale • Offer referral bonuses to existing employees

CONDUCTING EFFECTIVE INTERVIEWS

The goal when conducting interviews is to decide whether a job applicant is likely to be an excellent employee and a good fit for your practice. The biggest mistake managers make is being disorganized and unprepared. But those who adopt a strategic approach to job interviews and follow pre-determined protocols, maximize the chances of recruiting excellent team members. This is especially critical given the competitive job market in veterinary medicine. Managers need to be ready to act quickly to interview potential job candidates.

Before bringing job applicants in for interviews, decide on a defined protocol for the interview process. This includes making decisions about telephone interviews, use of job applications, deciding where to interview applicants, whether you will give a tour of the hospital, whether to do group or working interviews and last but not least how to avoid discrimination and adhere to legal guidelines. Let's take a look at some of these preparations.

Screening Candidates

One of the best ways to screen applicants is to conduct phone or virtual interviews using a platform such as zoom. Phone interviews are helpful if you have a large pool of applicants and need to narrow a list to the top candidates to offer in-person interviews. During phone interviews you can ask clarifying questions about skills and experience. This helps determine if the person is a good fit for your open position and culture. Phone interviews also provide information about a candidate's communication skills. If you're hiring a client service representative, phone interviews are an excellent way to hear how someone will sound to clients who call your practice. Some advantages of online interviews are that these meetings save time, eliminate travel costs, and you may be able to ascertain more about the candidate's level of interest in the position before bringing them in for an in-person interview.

Another way to screen applicants is to use job applications to gain relevant information and find out if someone has the qualifications for the job. Typically, job applications aren't used when interviewing veterinarians or managers, because practices have a small number of candidates who generally provide a resume or curriculum vitae. However, for hourly wage employees, job applications can be helpful as long as managers understand the need to avoid asking any illegal questions. As with in-person interviews, job applications should not include any questions that are discriminatory or prohibited by federal, state, or local laws. For example, many states now prohibit asking candidates about their criminal history. These are called "ban the box" laws.

Here are some questions included on job applications which provide insight about a potential employee that may not be included on their resume.

- Specific dates of employment. Sometimes people don't list dates on their resume and knowing this information may reveal if the candidate held a particular job for a brief period of time.
- The name of their supervisor and whether you may contact this former employer.
- The reason for leaving a job. This information helps you ask pertinent questions during the interview about what the candidate liked and didn't like about their previous job.
- The person's salary expectations. This can tell you if their desired salary is consistent with your pay range for the open position. Note, it is not acceptable to ask about salary history.
- What hours the person can work and when they can start work.

When screening candidates, be on the lookout for red flags that job applicants may not be a good fit for the practice or the job. Since finding qualified, talented team members is a challenge, it's easy to ignore these warning signs. But it doesn't make sense to waste valuable time interviewing someone who won't be a good addition to the team. Red flags may include having multiple jobs in a short period of time, resume spelling and grammar errors, unexplained gaps in employment, not including dates of employment, and not being available to work the required hours.

Lastly, it's a best practice to respond to all job applicants even those you don't grant an interview. Send an email thanking them for their interest in the position and letting them know their resume wasn't selected for further consideration. This helps convey a positive image for the practice and doesn't take much time if you use a template to cut and paste the appropriate response into an email.

Avoiding Discrimination

Take care to avoid discrimination throughout the entire recruitment and hiring process. For example, job ads should not include words that indicate the desire for a candidate of a certain age or gender. Ads should not reference any criteria that isn't related to doing the job and no job applicants should be eliminated from consideration for reasons such as their age, gender, sexual orientation, ethnicity, religion, or disability. One way to avoid bias is to define job qualifications for each position and decide what skills someone must have to be hired.

Avoid asking potential employees discriminatory and illegal questions. While job candidates may disclose personal information during an interview, refrain from continuing the conversation with illegal questions. For example, let's say someone mentions their children. It wouldn't be appropriate to then ask them how old their kids are or questions about their spouse. (See Figure Table 3.3: Legal vs. Illegal Interview Questions.)

Table 3.3: Legal vs. Illegal Interview Questions

Topic	Legal Questions	Illegal Questions
Personal	<ul><li>Do you have reliable transportation to work?</li><li>Do you have any responsibilities outside of work that would interfere with our job requirements?</li><li>What hours and days of the week can you work?</li></ul>	<ul><li>Are you married?</li><li>Do you have kids?</li><li>What do you do for childcare?</li><li>Do you own a car?</li><li>Do you own your house?</li></ul>
Religion	None	<ul><li>What church do you attend?</li><li>What religious holidays do you celebrate?</li></ul>
Citizenship	<ul><li>Are you legally eligible for employment in the U.S?</li></ul>	<ul><li>Where are you from?</li></ul>
Age	<ul><li>Are you 18 years of age or older?</li></ul>	<ul><li>How long have you been in the industry?</li><li>What is your age?</li><li>When did you graduate high school/college?</li></ul>
Disabilities	<ul><li>Can you perform all the duties of the job description for our open position?</li></ul>	<ul><li>Do you have disabilities?</li><li>Were you injured on the job?</li><li>Have you filed a Worker's Compensation claim before?</li></ul>

An excellent resource to find a list of legal vs. illegal interview questions is the Society for Human Resource Management (www.shrm.org). Educate everyone on your team about what questions to avoid. Many people will volunteer personal details about themselves especially during conversations they have with members of your team at their working interview. Just because you uncover these details, they should not factor into hiring decisions. It's discriminatory, for example, to decide not to hire someone because you think they're too old or have a young child that might get sick causing them to miss work.

Asking Effective Questions

Most employers conduct interviews in a business office at the practice. Regardless of where you conduct interviews, be sure the environment is consistent for all applicants and is as free from distractions as possible. Giving tours of the hospital before or after the formal interview is a best practice because it allows you the opportunity to showcase your practice and may stimulate questions from the candidate about the position.

Many practices conduct group or working interviews for the top candidates to gain more information about whether they have the requisite talent and skills for the job as well as whether they will be a good fit for the team. As with the rest of the interview process, be sure to standardize working interviews. Give every job applicant the same number of hours for the interview and try to have them meet with the same team members. You do need to investigate your state laws regarding compensation and liability concerns for working interviews. Be sure to clarify with both your team and the job applicant what they are allowed and not allowed to do during the working interview. It's also important to clearly communicate with the candidate if they will receive compensation for their time.

It's prudent to have a specific list of questions to ask all prospective employees which helps to avoid bias when making decisions about job fit and allows you to be able to make valid comparisons about candidates. Follow-up questions may be different for each interviewee, but use the same standard set of questions tailored for each position in the practice. Some questions may simply be to confirm or clarify information on a resume and job application. Other questions may be about the candidate's skills and qualifications. This includes questions such as "What practice management software system have you used?", "Tell me about your technical skills", and "What in-house laboratory equipment have you used?"

Otherwise, the best interview questions to ask are open-ended questions because they invite someone to give a more detailed response rather than saying "yes", "no" or a one-word response. For example, rather than asking "Did you like your last job" which could result in a yes/no response, a better question is to ask, "What did you like least about your last job?" which results in applicants giving you more information.

There are a limitless number of open-ended questions to ask, and many applicants are prepared for these questions.

Examples include:
- What did you like most or least about your last job?
- Describe your preferred work environment.
- What is your proudest accomplishment?
- Why do you want to work here?
- What are your strengths and what are your weaknesses?
- Tell me about your technical skills.

In addition to these types of questions, it's advisable to ask multiple behavioral based questions because they give you more insight about whether someone would be an excellent team member. There are two types of behavioral-based questions. The first is to present the candidate with a hypothetical scenario and ask how they would respond. For instance, you might describe a situation involving a lapse in client service and ask, "What would you do to calm an angry client?" This is a great question but recognize that a prepared candidate will reasonably know how to articulate a desired response.

The second type of behavioral based question is to ask the potential employee to tell you about situations involving their past jobs. These questions are effective because someone's past performance is most predictive of their future job performance. In this instance you would ask someone to tell you about a specific experience they've had interacting with an angry client or customer. You would change the question to "Tell me about a time when you were faced with an angry client. What happened and what did you do to calm the client?"

Don't worry if the applicant appears stumped and doesn't immediately answer a question. Just say "Take your time to think about my question" and avoid staring at them. If they still can't answer just say, "We can come back to this question later after you've had more time to think about it." Then you can see if the candidate volunteers an answer later in the interview and before concluding the interview, you can always offer them a second chance to respond.

Behavioral based questions help you gain more in-depth information about whether the potential employee will respond to work situations with behavior that aligns with your core values. Here are examples of several questions to ask related to the practice's core values:

For the core value *communication*:
- "Tell me about a situation where you failed to communicate appropriately. What would you have done differently?

For the core value *teamwork*:

- "Describe a time when you were a member of a team. What did you do to positively contribute to it?"

For the core value *compassionate care*:

- "Tell me about a time when you provided compassionate care to a pet."

There are 2 more keys to conducting effective interviews that will result in gaining the most knowledge about a job candidate. The first is to actively listen. Encourage potential employees to do most of the talking. By being a good listener and encouraging the candidate to speak freely, you learn more and may discover details about the person you didn't ask about.

The second key to your success is to ask follow-up open-ended questions after the prospective employee answers a question rather than just accepting every response at face value. This might include asking:

- "Can you give me an example of ……?"
- "Can you tell me more about what your thinking is on that?"
- "I'm not sure what you mean. Could you tell me more about that?"
- "You said you love client education. Can you describe how you find it best to educate clients?"

Before finishing an interview, it's a best practice to ask, "What questions do you have for me?" A well-prepared candidate will have several. In addition, take the opportunity to convey why the person would want to work at your hospital. In tight job markets, excellent job candidates likely have multiple interviews at area practices. Let them know why your business is an excellent choice for them. Include information about all benefits you offer as well as intangible rewards such as a great working environment with caring co-workers. And lastly, let interviewees know when you will get back with them. You don't want to leave someone hanging not knowing if they are a viable candidate and by the same token you don't want to lose out on hiring an outstanding team member because you were vague on when you would get back to someone about a working interview or a job offer. (See Figure 3.4: Effective Interview Questions for more examples of what to ask job candidates)

Table 3.4: Effective Interview Questions

Reason for questions	Questions to ask
To learn more about the candidate	• Tell me about your current/ recent job. Why do you want to make a change? • What are your goals and where do you want to be in the next 2 years? • What do you feel you need to be successful and happy in your job?
To assess job fit	• What do you think you will like most about this job? • How do you stay organized? • Describe your ideal work environment. What is your idea of a perfect workday or work week?
To assess alignment with culture and core values	• What are examples of how team members can show respect for one another? • How would you demonstrate compassion for a sick pet? • Tell me about one of your best success stories related to client education?
To assess interest in learning	• What are you better at today than you were this time last year? • Tell me something you don't know that you wished you did know? • What are your areas of interest and what skills would you like to improve on?
To verify competency and proficiency	• Which veins are you comfortable doing venipuncture on? • How many IV catheters have you routinely placed each day? • What types of digital communications did you use at your last job? • What client education topics are you comfortable discussing with pet owners?
To predict future behavior	• Tell me about a time when you were part of a team that was struggling. What happened and what was the outcome? • Tell me about a time when a client or customer was upset about a wrong charge or their bill. What happened and what did you do? • Tell me about a time when you worked with someone you didn't like or who was unkind to you. How did you handle the situation?

EVALUATING CANDIDATES AND MAKING JOB OFFERS

After concluding each interview, it's beneficial to evaluate and rank the job candidate while the interview is fresh in your mind. Evaluation forms can be used to help assess everyone fairly and consistently. Typically, applicants are rated in the areas of technical skills, knowledge, specific work experience, interpersonal and communication skills, alignment with core values and professionalism. Be mindful to avoid any unconscious bias when assessing job fit and/or comparing applicants. Additionally, one of the best ways to fairly evaluate candidates is to consider before the interview what responses you want to hear that will indicate someone is a good fit for the position and most likely to be able to competently perform their job duties. For example, let's say you're hiring a veterinary assistant and ask them "why do you want to work here?" You want to hear them say that they value helping pets and people not just that they love animals and/or need a full-time job.

The next step is to check references for any candidate you're considering hiring. While checking references can be time consuming, you may not obtain the information you seek, and positive references don't guarantee new employees will work out, savvy managers know it's an integral part of successful recruitment. Checking references serves 2 basic purposes. One is to verify factual information such as dates of employment and job duties. The other is to inquire about the candidate's work experience and personal attributes to ascertain if they are qualified and likely to be a good team member.

Most resumes either list references or state "references available upon request." It's safe to assume the references provided by someone seeking a job are going to be positive. So, calling these references may not be fruitful unless it includes former employers or co-workers. The best references to call are supervisors or owners of the business where the job applicant has worked who can answer specific questions about the person's job performance.

Before we review what questions to ask, let's look at problems you may run into when calling references. The first is many businesses, especially larger corporations, won't release any information other than dates of employment. Even if you get the candidate's manager on the phone, they may decline to give information and refer you to the HR department. You may also run into situations where the person's previous manager is no longer with the company. If this happens, ask the prospective employee for the names of other supervisors or co-workers who can serve as references. Another problem occurs when the job applicant is still working and doesn't want you to contact their current employer who doesn't know they are job hunting. In this instance, you have to assess if the reason for wanting to leave their current position seems valid. Ultimately, if there is limited information from references, managers may have to rely solely on their evaluation of the candidate.

To get the most out of calls to references, be prepared with a set of questions. To begin the call identify yourself, state the purpose of your call, and tell the reference what position their former employee will be filling. Then ask easy questions such as verifying dates of employment and assigned job duties. Clarify whether the reference has first-hand knowledge of the job candidate's work and how long they worked with them. A reference from a direct supervisor carries more weight than one from a manager in another department.

Sometimes, previous employers readily volunteer substantial information about the candidate. Usually this happens because the employee was an excellent team member and they're eager to help them get another job. You may find yourself listening to a list of reasons why you should hire this person. Be careful this doesn't distract you from getting the answers to the questions you prepared. You don't want to miss relevant details about prior work experience just because you're excited about the positive reference.

Here are examples of excellent questions to ask job references:

- Can you tell me about the level of proficiency of her/his technical skills?
- Was the employee punctual? Were there any issues with tardiness or absenteeism?
- Did he/she receive any promotions or demotions, or remain in the same role throughout their tenure?
- Did they go beyond what was required without being asked?
- Ask for specific examples of how the employee did their job that relate to your core values such as "what's an example of Lisa's commitment to teamwork?" or "Can you tell me about how Lisa likes to educate pet owners?"
- What roles and/or additional responsibilities did the employee have?
- Is there anything else I should take into consideration before I hire this candidate?

If a former employer seems reluctant to say much, this may be an indication they had problems with the employee, and you need to ask the right questions to glean this information. One question that needs to be on your list is to ask whether the candidate is eligible for rehire. Of course, if the employer says "no", they wouldn't rehire the candidate, you can follow up with the questions of "Why not?" and "What was his or her reason for leaving?" Be patient at this point in the conversation because most people don't want to give negative feedback that hurts someone's chance of gaining employment and they may be concerned about liability. It can be helpful to give some details about what type of employee you're looking for and volunteer if you noted anything in the interview that raised a red flag. Sometimes when you open up, the former employer will open up or at least validate that your concerns are well founded.

After checking references and rating job candidates, it's time to decide if you want to offer a job to any of your applicants and if so to whom. Most managers don't have a problem narrowing the list of qualified applicants to a few top candidates. At this point, any numerical ranking or rating of the potential employees is likely to be close. While gut instincts are not without merit, now is not the time to abandon your strategic approach to recruitment.

Here are the factors to consider when comparing job applicants.

- Who has the highest skill level?
- Who has the best soft skills based on responses to interview questions?
- Who seems to be the best fit for your team? Who does the team give the highest rating?
- Any budget considerations

When making a job offer, it's best to give potential employees a written summary of compensation, benefits, and the value of joining the practice. In addition to stating wages, include the dollar value of all benefits and specifics about intangibles such as positive aspects of the practice culture. After talking to the job applicant, you can email the job offer as a pdf on the company letterhead. First, this helps to avoid any misunderstandings about salary, benefits, and job expectations. Second, it sends a clear, professional message that the business is serious and excited about having the job applicant join the practice. And lastly, it gives the potential employee written information about why they should join the team.

SUMMARY

Successful recruitment hinges on having a defined system in place with specific protocols so it's easy to act when the need arises to hire a new employee. Managers that engage in proper planning and organization are best positioned to recruit and hire qualified, productive team members who will contribute to the success of the practice. Since recruitment in veterinary medicine is competitive, the practice needs on-going efforts aimed at becoming a preferred employer so the business can convey to potential new hires the "what's in it for me" (WIFM). And lastly, given the shortage of job candidates, it's wise to extend job offers quickly if managers find someone they like because most qualified applicants will have multiple offers.

CHAPTER 4

Team Training

The practice needs fully trained team members to consistently deliver high-quality medical care to patients and exceptional service to pet owners. The goal of a successful training program is to make sure the entire team receives sufficient training so they can be proficient at their jobs. Not just a few people, but everyone. Not just some of the time, but all the time. Trained teams possess the relevant knowledge, skills, and competencies they need to be efficient and productive. When the practice has an effective training program, employee job satisfaction and morale improves, team members are able to utilize their skills to their maximum potential, patient care and client care are optimal, and the business is more successful.

The amount of training required for employees to become proficient at their jobs can be extensive. Understandably, managers may feel overwhelmed trying to implement a comprehensive training program for the practice. Here are common obstacles and challenges managers face:

- Lack of time for training
- Staff shortages and/or not enough experienced employees to train their co-workers
- The need to create and provide comprehensive training programs for the entire team
- Developing a training program with sufficient tools and resources
- Lack of clarity about gaps in training
- Unrealistic expectations or a lack of understanding for how long it takes employees to learn
- Team members who see training as a burden and resent having to train new hires
- Team members who are reluctant to share knowledge with co-workers
- Failure to delegate and empower employees to train new hires or their peers

If any of those challenges sound familiar, then this chapter will help you get organized and take the necessary steps to implement a training program for both new hires and current team members. Remember, veterinary medicine is always changing; there is always something new to learn. For training to be effective, the practice culture needs to promote continuous learning. Go back to your core values and their descriptors. Do you have core values such as "innovation", "excellence" or "knowledge"? Is life-long learning mentioned? Does the practice's devotion to excellence reference the need to be progressive and provide cutting-edge medical care? Do your core values mention advancing the team's knowledge and education so they can provide the highest quality care? What about staying current with new protocols to provide a high standard of care?

Practices that do a good job with training have systems in place to deliver training, involve the entire team, and are proud of their dedication to continuous learning. It isn't easy to be one of those practices because it takes time and a commitment to training that never ends. There will always be employee turnover leading to new hires who need training. Team members will always need on-going training related to new products, services, procedures, protocols, diseases, and medical conditions. If you already have a robust training program, you can use this chapter as a checklist to see if you need to enhance or modify your system. If your training program is a work in progress, you can use the information here to create an action plan to achieve your goals.

EMPLOYEE ORIENTATION

Training begins with employee orientation which is the process of introducing new employees to their jobs and the workplace. The purpose of orientation for new hires is to help them integrate into the company so they can be successful. Part of the orientation process is to help make people feel welcome and valued as a new team member. Not only does this benefit new hires, but studies show that orientation programs help increase employee retention for the business.[1] Company studies have also shown that employees who go through detailed orientation are more productive sooner than employees who don't go through the program.[2] Despite the proven benefits of employee orientation, veterinary practices don't always have a formal orientation process or if they do, it is so brief as to be ineffective.

The best way to organize a complete orientation program is to create a detailed checklist that outlines all the relevant activities for the orientation process (see Figure 4.1 for an orientation checklist). This ensures you obtain relevant information the business needs from new hires and that employees receive the information they need to be successful. You can divide the checklist into categories such as new hire paperwork, a review of benefits, job duties, practice policies, hospital procedures, and introductions. Note that it is advisable for the checklist to include having a supervisor or manager explain the introductory period to let new hires know when to expect an employee review during this time. Another critical part of orientation is to include action steps for how new hires will gain knowledge about the practice history, mission, vision, core values and culture. The goal is for new employees to gain an understanding of what it means to work at the practice and how they fit in.

As stated previously, orientation periods are often way too short. When practices experience staff shortages, it's tempting to have newly hired employees hit the ground running as quickly as possible. Unfortunately, when his happens people can easily become frustrated trying to absorb so much new information or complete job duties without sufficient training. To avoid this pitfall, create a realistic orientation schedule that spreads items on the checklist over a period of one or more weeks. And don't forget to establish who will meet with employees during the orientation period. The last thing a new employee (or manager) wants to hear from a co-worker is "I didn't know I was supposed to meet with Sally. I don't have time for that!"

Perhaps the most overlooked aspect of employee orientation is to make it as enjoyable as possible for the entire team and to make new hires feel welcome. The orientation process starts before the employee's first day of employment, so they walk in knowing what to expect and excited to come to their new job. You can email the orientation schedule to new employees, so they know how they'll spend their time the first day and the first week. Let new team members know they will need to fill out paperwork and advise them to bring any necessary documents. As part of their paperwork, consider having new hires fill out a survey to gain more information about their interests and how they like to receive recognition (see Figure 4.2 for a sample new hire survey.) Another welcoming gesture is to personally call new hires a day or two before they start to see if they have any questions. It's also a good idea to tell them who will greet them when they arrive for work.

The first day of a new job can be nerve-wracking for some people. To put new hires at ease, make sure everyone on the team knows when a new employee is coming to work and their role in welcoming them. You can make assignments, for example, for specific team members to give the new hire a tour of the building, sit with them if they eat lunch at the hospital, and be their guide for the first day. Don't forget to include the practice owner and associate veterinarians in orientation.

Figure 4.1 New Hire Orientation Checklist

New Hire Orientation Checklist

Employee Name: _____

Welcome
- _____ Inform team of new hire start date
- _____ Send welcome email to new hire
- _____ Call 2 days prior to start date: see if new hire has questions and convey relevant reminders
- _____ Prepare welcome gift for first day
- _____ Assign orientation guide and/or mentor
- _____ Schedule team "Get to know you" activities for the first week of employment

Team introductions
- _____ Tour hospital; where to put personal belongings, break room
- _____ Meet and greet with all team members
- _____ Introduce to orientation guide/trainer/supervisor
- _____ Introduce to "lunch buddy" for first day if employee stays at hospital for lunch
- _____ Meeting with practice owner to review hospital history, philosophy, and vision
- _____ Meeting with manager to review mission, core values and culture

New hire paperwork
- _____ Personal contact information
- _____ W-4 Form
- _____ I-9 Form
- _____ Benefits forms for health insurance and retirement plans
- _____ State income tax withholding forms
- _____ Copy of state license or certification (for DVMs, credentialed technicians)
- _____ Fill out new hire survey

Review of benefits
- _____ Review all hospital provided insurance benefits
- _____ Review hospital retirement plan
- _____ Explain personal pet healthcare benefits
- _____ Explain employee assistance program (EAP)
- _____ Review time off policy (PTO, sick days, vacation days, holidays)
- _____ Review pay schedule, uniform allowance, CE allowance

Review job duties
- _____ Review job description, job roles and job expectations
- _____ Review end of day and other work checklists
- _____ Review work schedule
- _____ Know how to access work schedules

Figure 4.1 New Hire Orientation Checklist (continued)

Review hospital policies, SOPs, and operations
_____ Review employee manual and sign acknowledgement of receipt
_____ Review introductory period expectations and timing for reviews
_____ Show how to clock in and complete time sheets for each pay period
_____ Locate fire extinguishers and emergency exits
_____ Know the location of emergency eye wash station (s)
_____ Learn medical waste disposal procedures
_____ Show location of binders and digital file folders for hospital SOPs, protocols, and training guides

Figure 4.2 New Hire Survey

New Hire Survey

Please let us know your primary areas of interest and any projects or assignments you may be willing to assist with.

- ☐ Feline medicine
- ☐ Behavior
- ☐ Dentistry
- ☐ Preventive care plans for clients
- ☐ Learning more about pet nutrition
- ☐ Pet obesity program
- ☐ Helping with Cat Friendly or Fear Free initiatives
- ☐ Client communications
- ☐ Surgery
- ☐ Pain management
- ☐ Laser therapy and rehab
- ☐ Senior care program
- ☐ Puppy/kitten kits
- ☐ Puppy training/kitten socialization
- ☐ Digital client communications/Social media posts
- ☐ Helping organize community events
- ☐ Team building events
- ☐ Party planning ideas
- ☐ Other: _____

Check the boxes for activities you enjoy that we might be able to do as a team

- ☐ Bowling
- ☐ Paint ball
- ☐ Wall climbing
- ☐ Hiking
- ☐ Watching football
- ☐ Baseball games
- ☐ Miniature golf
- ☐ BBQ or anything that involves food!
- ☐ Walking
- ☐ Laser tag
- ☐ TopGolf
- ☐ City sightseeing
- ☐ Kayaking
- ☐ Scavenger hunts
- ☐ Board games
- ☐ Crafts
- ☐ Escape room
- ☐ Cooking classes
- ☐ Painting classes
- ☐ Trivia
- ☐ Movies
- ☐ Community volunteer work
- ☐ Dog or cat shows
- ☐ Other_____

How do you like to receive recognition or rewards? (Check all that apply)

- ☐ Public verbal words of appreciation
- ☐ Acknowledgement privately
- ☐ Recognition at team meeting
- ☐ Thank you cards
- ☐ Gift cards
- ☐ Recognition on social media
- ☐ Award or gift as a token of appreciation
- ☐ Additional paid time off

Busy veterinarians (or any team member) might come across as intimidating so be sure everyone understands the value of making a point to welcome new team members on their first day. Ideally, the practice owner(s) or medical director should meet with new hires to personally explain the practice's history, philosophy, and culture. This demonstrates interest and respect towards the new employee and allows them to hear firsthand about the passions of the practice owner and the history of the business.

Welcome gifts are always well-received and don't have to be expensive. For example, you can fill a coffee mug with items such as pens, magnets, a pet bandana, snack bars and candy. Other ideas include a small cactus, gift card, or movie passes. During the first week of employment, try to make time for several interactive team exercises that help new hires get to know their co-workers. These sessions can be short standing meetings held right before lunch or another convenient time. You might put interesting and fun questions in a bowl and have everyone take turns answering questions such as "Would you rather be a groundhog or a fox?" and "If you could teleport yourself anywhere, where would it be?" These types of exercises are fun for everyone and don't put the new hire on the spot or make them the center of attention.

SUCCESSFULLY ON-BOARDING NEW HIRES

On-boarding is the process of helping a new employee integrate into the business and gain the skills, knowledge, and competencies they need to become a productive team member. It is not the same as orientation although orientation is part of the on-boarding process.[3] Effective on-boarding involves making sure employees receive initial training to do their job as well as all the training, tools and support they need to become proficient in their job roles. Depending on their level of ability when hired, the on-boarding process may take up to a full year. At a minimum, think of the 90-day introductory period as an employee's time for on-boarding.

As with orientation, effective on-boarding helps to enhance employee retention. You can find numerous statistics on the internet touting the benefits of having an outstanding on-boarding program as a means to retain top talent and reduce employee turnover. Which only makes sense because no one wants to struggle trying to do their job. Successfully on-boarding new hires also helps boost team morale because no one wants to work with a co-worker who isn't trained to do their job.

Despite the fact that many practices routinely experience challenges related to staff shortages, it's not uncommon for employees to express frustration at having to train new hires. Understandably, having to provide instruction to new co-workers can slow down workflow and add stress during the day for trainers. To minimize the burden on any one person, if possible, try to divide training duties among multiple team members during each day. For example, when onboarding CSRs, one employee can spend a few hours training them on answering phones, a different employee can spend a few hours teaching them how to use the practice management software, and a technician can schedule time with them to explain preventive care standards.

For on-boarding new employees to work well, you need a detailed plan that includes timelines because without structure, the on-boarding process falls apart. On-boarding plans should outline what new hires need to learn and be able to do each week the first one to two months and then monthly thereafter. (For an example of a technician/assistant onboarding checklist and a training checklist, see Figures 4.3 and 4.4.) In addition, on-boarding should include feedback and review sessions with a manager as well as assessment tools to ensure team members retain information and gain the requisite proficiency needed to fully contribute to the practice. In the next sections of this chapter, you will find details on how to implement hospital training programs to support your on-boarding plan.

As noted in chapter three, mentorship programs are a good way to build your hospital's reputation and recruit team members. Moreover, mentors can help with on-boarding new hires. Mentorship is particularly valuable when on-boarding newly graduated veterinarians. But mentors can help any new employee successfully integrate into the practice and make sure they have the tools they need to excel. Bear in mind not all experienced employees are necessarily good mentors. Some people don't have the patience or willingness to mentor their co-workers. For those team members who are willing to be mentors, it's critical for the practice to provide guidance and training so they know how to best help their mentees. This includes clarifying expectations for both mentors and mentees, setting up a schedule for meetings, establishing goals for mentees, and making sure mentors know how to engage mentees with questions.

Team Training

Figure 4.3 Technician/assistant Onboarding Checklist

Technician/Assistant On-boarding Checklist

Employee Name: _____

(Supervisor, trainer, or team lead to initial upon each completion of a skill or task)

Hospital operations
- _____ _____ Locate the SDS for common chemicals
- _____ _____ Know location of drugs and supplies for emergencies
- _____ _____ Know how to access team meeting summaries
- _____ _____ Know medication refill protocols
- _____ _____ Learn how to prepare and label medications for dispensing
- _____ _____ Learn how to fill out paperwork to request lab tests
- _____ _____ Learn how to check/print/log/alert doctors about lab results
- _____ _____ Learn exam room protocols

Learn how to use Practice Information Management Software (PIMS):
- _____ _____ Enter a new client
- _____ _____ Enter a new patient
- _____ _____ Make an appointment
- _____ _____ Learn appointment protocols
- _____ _____ Enter information into physical exam sheet or medical plan/synopsis
- _____ _____ Enter/update patient reminders
- _____ _____ Record a client phone call conversation or message

Learn process for patient admission to hospital
- _____ _____ Review medical record to confirm client and patient information
- _____ _____ Ask appropriate questions and confirm services due
- _____ _____ Make sure check in form signed (anesthesia/client treatment form)
- _____ _____ Get a current weight for patient
- _____ _____ Set up patient identification (e.g. cage card, collar tag)
- _____ _____ Enter patient on the whiteboard/initiate a medical plan/enter medical notes
- _____ _____ Communicating relevant information to co-workers
- _____ _____ Alerting doctor about patient and client needs

Client Communications
- _____ _____ Learn puppy/kitten vaccination and testing protocols
- _____ _____ Learn canine/feline adult vaccination and testing protocols
- _____ _____ Know features and benefits of heartworm, flea/tick products
- _____ _____ Learn hospital standards for how to properly answer phone and greet clients
- _____ _____ Know and understand usage of hospital app and digital client communications
- _____ _____ Know common medical abbreviations
- _____ _____ Understand basic medical terminology

Figure 4.4 Technician/assistant Training Checklist

Technician/Assistant Training Checklist

Name_____

(Doctor, supervisor, trainer, or team lead to initial upon each completion of a skill or task)

Client Communications
- ___ ___ ___ Instruct clients on proper feeding of therapeutic diets
- ___ ___ ___ Client education on administration of insulin, signs to monitor
- ___ ___ ___ Client discharge instructions for post-op procedures and dentistry
- ___ ___ ___ Know how to explain and present payment options

Patient Care
- ___ ___ ___ Properly clean and disinfect cages
- ___ ___ ___ Prepare meals for hospitalized patients
- ___ ___ ___ Properly sanitize food and water bowls
- ___ ___ ___ Restrain animals correctly for all procedures
- ___ ___ ___ Remove frightened animals from cages or run
- ___ ___ ___ Apply a muzzle
- ___ ___ ___ Trim nails
- ___ ___ ___ Clean ears
- ___ ___ ___ Express anal glands
- ___ ___ ___ Properly trim hair for a potty path
- ___ ___ ___ Properly administer subcutaneous fluids

Patient Care
- ___ ___ ___ Prepare IV fluids and a catheter for use
- ___ ___ ___ Flush IV catheters and change iv fluid bags
- ___ ___ ___ Place an IV catheter
- ___ ___ ___ Place feline IV catheter
- ___ ___ ___ Place an IV catheter in a brachycephalic breed (e.g., Dachshund, Bassett)
- ___ ___ ___ Place IV catheter in puppy/kitten
- ___ ___ ___ Properly add medication to an IV bag/label bag
- ___ ___ ___ Administer an IV injection
- ___ ___ ___ Administer a SQ injection
- ___ ___ ___ Administer an IM injection

CBC
- ___ ___ ___ Know preparation and samples needed to complete test
- ___ ___ ___ Be familiar with maintenance
- ___ ___ ___ Learn how to run a CBC

Serum chemistries analyzer
- ___ ___ ___ Know what tests machine runs
- ___ ___ ___ Know preparation and samples needed to complete each test
- ___ ___ ___ Be familiar with maintenance

UA Machine
- ___ ___ ___ Learn how to prepare a urine strip
- ___ ___ ___ Learn how to correctly calibrate machine

Refractometer
- ___ ___ ___ Become familiar with proper storage of the refractometer

Figure 4.4 Technician/assistant Training Checklist (continued)

_____ _____ _____ Become familiar with using/reading the refractometer
_____ _____ _____ Know proper cleaning of the refractometer

Learn how to collect urine and properly perform a complete urinalysis:
_____ _____ _____ Cystocentesis
_____ _____ _____ Free Catch
_____ _____ _____ Specific Gravity
_____ _____ _____ Urine Strip
_____ _____ _____ Sediment
_____ _____ _____ Record results

Learn how to prepare samples and complete in-house lab testing
_____ _____ _____ Learn how to log/send out/prepare samples for reference lab testing
_____ _____ _____ Check/print/log lab results
_____ _____ _____ FELV/FIV Test
_____ _____ _____ Parvo Test
_____ _____ _____ PCV
_____ _____ _____ TP
_____ _____ _____ Glucose

Centrifuge
_____ _____ _____ Learn how to properly balance machine
_____ _____ _____ Learn settings
_____ _____ _____ Learn which vials/tests can be spun in centrifuge

Microscope
_____ _____ _____ Become familiar with each power objectives
_____ _____ _____ Know what power to use on each test
_____ _____ _____ Learn how to properly clean microscope
_____ _____ _____ Learn how to perform ear cytology
_____ _____ _____ Learn how to perform a skin scrape
_____ _____ _____ Learn how to perform skin cytology
_____ _____ _____ Learn how to perform a heartworm microfilaria test
_____ _____ _____ Properly prepare and read fecals

Radiology
_____ _____ _____ Turn on/off machine
_____ _____ _____ Request images
_____ _____ _____ Use of personal protection equipment
_____ _____ _____ Use of collimator
_____ _____ _____ How to read the measuring chart
_____ _____ _____ Capture images

Dental radiology
_____ _____ _____ Understand cat/dog dental charts
_____ _____ _____ Learn how to properly perform feline oral rads
_____ _____ _____ Learn how to properly perform canine oral rads
_____ _____ _____ Know proper grading of gingivitis and dental disease

Doppler/ECG
_____ _____ _____ Be familiar with and learn troubleshooting techniques for each instrument
_____ _____ _____ Become familiar with proper blood pressure cuff measuring/use
_____ _____ _____ Become familiar with the supplies needed to perform a Doppler blood pressure

Figure 4.4 Technician/assistant Training Checklist (continued)

_____ _____ _____ Become familiar with proper storage of Doppler
_____ _____ _____ Learn what to use to clean each instrument
_____ _____ _____ Become familiar with "normal" values for each instrument
_____ _____ _____ Properly perform an ECG
_____ _____ _____ Properly perform a Doppler blood pressure measurement

Ultrasonic Cleaner

_____ _____ _____ Learn what solution to use for ultrasonic cleaner
_____ _____ _____ Learn how to properly fill ultrasonic cleaner
_____ _____ _____ Learn how to properly run ultrasonic cleaner
_____ _____ _____ Become familiar with maintenance

Autoclave/instrument packs

_____ _____ _____ Learn how to properly fill autoclave
_____ _____ _____ Become familiar with each cycle
_____ _____ _____ Become familiar with maintenance
_____ _____ _____ Learn to identify and care for common instruments
_____ _____ _____ Learn how to properly prepare and sterilize surgical packs:
_____ _____ _____ General and specific instrument packs
_____ _____ _____ Gown packs
_____ _____ _____ Towel/drape packs
_____ _____ _____ Eye pack
_____ _____ _____ Cold sterilization

Ultrasound

_____ _____ _____ Able to turn the ultrasound on/off
_____ _____ _____ Become familiar with proper storage of the probe

Surgery

_____ _____ _____ Learn anesthesia protocols
_____ _____ _____ identify stages and planes of anesthesia
_____ _____ _____ Understand anesthesia machines
_____ _____ _____ Know how to properly monitor anesthetized patients
_____ _____ _____ Administer anesthetics
_____ _____ _____ Intubate dogs
_____ _____ _____ Intubate cats
_____ _____ _____ Prepare patients for surgery
_____ _____ _____ Setup for a surgery
_____ _____ _____ Setup for a dental
_____ _____ _____ Setup for prepping a surgery

Learn how to assist with following surgeries and procedures: (E.g., check in patient, setup surgery suite, instruments and packs needed, administer anesthesia, prep patient, patient monitoring, extubate, post-surgery care, enter client charges, post-op client instructions, discharge procedures)

_____ _____ _____ Spay
_____ _____ _____ Neuter
_____ _____ _____ Dentistry procedures
_____ _____ _____ Mass Removal
_____ _____ _____ Blocked Cat
_____ _____ _____ Abdominal surgery
_____ _____ _____ Lacerations or wound care

SETTING UP EFFECTIVE TRAINING PROGRAMS

As noted earlier, the goal of an employee training program is to provide sufficient education so everyone on the team has the knowledge, skills, and abilities to do their job competently. To achieve this goal, practices need an organized program that is comprehensive in scope such that it supports training for new hires as well as on-going training for current employees to consistently enhance their knowledge and skills. Successful training programs have multiple modules that collectively provide the structure and necessary resources for all employees in the company to learn and grow. Given the magnitude of creating and implementing such a complete training system, multiple team members need to participate in the process. It isn't realistic or reasonable for managers to shoulder the responsibility for the practice's entire training program without assistance from other employees and outside parties.

One of the best ways to build an effective training program is to create a training team comprised of three to six people representing all departments in the hospital. You may have difficulty finding people who want to be on the team. To overcome this obstacle, it's essential to emphasize the benefits of having a comprehensive training program. Most team members appreciate the frustration of working with an untrained co-worker, so that alone may motivate them to be a part of the training team. In addition to the benefits of improved teamwork and productivity, remind employees how team training improves patient and client care. This is a good time to reference the core values of the practice. The idea is to get reluctant employees to see that helping with training isn't just a task they must complete, but rather a valuable activity that helps more pets get care they deserve.

Be sure to clearly define the training team's roles, responsibilities, and job expectations. (See Figure 4.5 Training Team Roles.) Of course, for a training team to be successful, they need time allocated to complete work and hold meetings to discuss their progress. Training teams work most efficiently when they're given direction and empowered to reach established goals. During the team's first meeting managers can create dialogue to explore ideas about how to meet the goals. There are no right or wrong approaches for how managers work with training teams. Sometimes managers complete the lion's share of work and in other instances, the training team functions with minimal oversight from the manager. Just remember, teams are more likely to perform at a higher level when you delegate a specific amount of work, set up deadlines, and reward the team for their efforts. Rewards may be in the form of praise, thank-you cards, gift cards, or bonuses, just to name a few.

Figure 4.5 Training Team Roles

Training Team Roles

Oversight and direction of team: _____

Team members: _____

Team Goal: Create and implement a comprehensive training program for both new hires and existing team members.

Job roles and responsibilities

- Create a list of training topics for technicians, assistants, client service representatives (CSRs).
- Edit and/or draft training documents, e.g., checklists, protocols, how to guides, instructions.
- Identify outside training resources, e.g., webinars, videos, lunch and learns by vendors, articles.
- Organize training materials into notebooks or folders as well as digital files.
- Provide one-on-one or group training to co-workers as assigned and agreed upon.
- Create timelines & deadlines for assignments.
- Hold each other accountable to completing assignments.
- Be an advocate for training and learning; be a role model and cheerleader.
- Demonstrate patience as co-workers learn; stay positive and encourage co-workers.
- Understand people learn at different paces and in different ways so a one size fits all approach may not work.
- Solicit feedback from co-workers regarding their challenges and progress.
- Solicit feedback from veterinarians and supervisors regarding gaps in training and progress of team members.
- Use a system to keep track of training needs and requests, e.g., a notebook used by all team members kept in central location and/or a suggestion box for the team.
- Act as liaisons for communication between departments.
- Identify problems or areas needing improvement and propose solutions.
- Proposed solutions must meet with approval of management.
- Submit requests for any required resources to management.

Job expectations

- Meet as a team monthly at a minimum; meet in smaller groups weekly or biweekly.
- Designate one person to lead each all-team meeting.
- Type minutes into Word document during meetings; place in Training Team notebook and digital file.
- Stay focused to allow time for discussion as well as problem solving.
- Schedule meetings to minimize interference with the efficiency and operations of the hospital.
- Communicate with each other, co-workers, and upper management in a respectful and positive manner.
- Create a clear action plan with deadlines at every meeting. Focus efforts on a few items at a time to be most successful.

Even with careful planning and organization, managers may face difficulties when implementing comprehensive training programs. Here are training challenges to be aware of:

- Failure to establish training objectives and a schedule for learning
- Going too fast for employees who need a slower pace for learning
- Not prioritizing basic job tasks and knowledge before moving to advanced knowledge and skills
- Trainers are too busy to train well; failure to adjust work schedules to allow time for training
- The training process is too passive, e.g., employees only observe co-workers before they're expected to complete job tasks on their own
- Programs with insufficient supporting tools or resources, e.g., auditory instruction alone
- On the job training without any measurements of retention of knowledge

To avoid some of these problems, create a written training plan and use a checklist (see checklist in Figure 4.6). Note that the checklist should include a timeline and schedule for all training programs as well as the need to evaluate the program at least annually.

Figure 4.6: Checklist to Implement an Effective Training Program

Checklist to Implement an Effective Training Program

1. Work with team members to identify a list of all training topics and goals for each training module. (E.g., client communications, basic animal restraint, lab procedures, exam room procedures, etc.)
2. Identify and prioritize training needs for each department.
3. Utilize orientation and training checklists to track each team member's progress.
4. Make assignments: who will provide training on each topic and when. (Team members who aren't on the training team can do some of the training)
5. Identify training resources such as:
    a. Courses offered by professional organizations, e.g., AAHA, AVMA, VHMA
    b. Training resources provided by pharmaceutical companies, petfood companies and distributors
    c. In-house education from veterinarians
    d. Lunch and learns from vendors
    e. Relevant articles and case studies
6. Use resources to assess retention of information learned such as:
    a. Quizzes
    b. Checklists
    c. Practical exams to evaluate proficiency
    d. Interactive communications skills training
    e. Oral exams
7. Identify and brainstorm solutions for the following barriers to training:
    a. Time constraints
    b. Communication breakdowns
    c. Lack of cooperation from team members
    d. Doctors or other team members undermining training efforts
    e. Not having programs that adapt to various learning styles
    f. Figure 4.6: Checklist to Implement an Effective Training Program (continued)
8. Organize and create structure for the training program:
    a. How to keep track of documents: e.g., notebooks and digital file folders
    b. Create a library of resources by topic area
    c. Give each team member a pocket folder to organize their training documents
9. Create timeline and deadlines for work assignments.
10. Evaluate the program quarterly.

Once the practice has an organized plan and training team in place, the next step is to complete a needs assessment to uncover gaps in training. For example, perhaps the practice has an excellent education program for client service representatives, but it doesn't include phone skills training. Or maybe the practice needs to provide more instruction for technicians in the areas of anesthesia and patient monitoring. You can use employee job descriptions as the foundation to determine training needs. Logically, the practice needs some form of training for team members to be proficient completing all their job duties. In addition, employees need training in other areas such as OSHA compliance, well-being, diversity and inclusion, conflict management skills, and understanding all the hospital protocols. The team also needs training when new products and services are introduced in the hospital. This might include training on the features and benefits of a new preventive product or how to provide (or assist with) new services such as laser therapy.

The most successful training programs afford employees in each department the opportunity to attain higher levels of proficiency and learn more advanced skills. Practices with outstanding training programs often implement what is termed levels or phased training. With this type of training, employees can progress to a higher level in their job position (and often higher wage) by gaining more knowledge and skills. For example, you may have three or four levels for veterinary assistants with the lowest level being inexperienced, new hires and the highest-level assistants having skills similar to credentialed veterinary technicians. Make sure the practice has clear distinctions for each level, proposed timelines for employees to move from one level to the next, clear expectations about wage increases, and designated trainers for each phase of the training program. Bear in mind job duties performed by veterinary assistants and credentialed technicians must be in accordance with your state's veterinary medicine practice act.

How To Handle Time Constraints

The number one reason practice managers and team members alike cite for not having everyone trained is a lack of time. This is a challenge for busy practices, and it is exacerbated when teams are short-staffed. In Chapter 1, you learned that being a productive manager requires effective time management. To implement successful training programs, you will need to devote time to planning, organization, and scheduling of training sessions. Half the battle to deal with time constraints is to have a comprehensive, organized program in place with tools and resources because this creates greater efficiency. You have a plan ready to go anytime there is a training need. The other half is making time in the schedule on a regular basis for employees to engage in training and learning.

Decide on ideal times for training. Many practices find it works well to complete training mid-day during the lunch break. This is a suitable time to have company representatives conduct monthly lunch 'n learns for the entire team or to facilitate in-house training. You can also devote thirty minutes of the lunch break once or twice a week to a training session. Another strategy is to put 20-30 minute time blocks somewhere in the work schedule a few times a week for specific employees to engage in learning. Team members can use designated times to watch short videos, read articles, take quizzes, or meet with a trainer to practice new skills.

An often-overlooked strategy is to shorten the time increments for training so they're easier to schedule. One way to do this is to hold standing meetings that last about fifteen minutes. Typically standing meetings involve a smaller group of team members. These meetings work well because they tend to be more interactive and require minimal advance planning. Standing meetings are an excellent way for team members to engage with one another as they learn. Veterinarians, credentialed technicians, or managers can provide training during these sessions on topics such as client communication skills, parasite prevention, features of new products, and using low stress patient handling techniques.

Another strategy is to narrow the goals and action steps for training. Focus on one skill or topic area at a time. Rather than trying to teach a veterinary assistant four new skills, concentrate on one at a time. A team member might, for example, focus solely on learning exam room client communications for two or more weeks. This doesn't mean someone can't learn multiple skills at a time, but trainers should emphasize the highest priority skills first. And of course, take advantage of slow times by having training sessions as the go-to activity rather than other less important job tasks.

Resources For Training

As you create, organize, and enhance your hospital's training program, consider what type of resources will make it more effective. Think of three types of resources: ones that assist with organization, tools that help facilitate learning, and resources that help measure retention of knowledge or proficiency of a skill. Determine what resources the practice already has available and what tools or resources you (or the training team) needs to find to support your program. The team may be able to create some training tools and they can identify outside resources available for purchase. There are a variety of companies that offer veterinary training tools, webinars, videos, training modules, courses, and subscription based learning services. Decide what resources are best for each component of your hospital's training program.

Resources for organization includes written schedules that outline time frames for training and checklists that help people track their progress. For example, new hires should have an on-boarding training schedule for the first 90 days of employment, and it should specify what tools are available to employees for each part of their training. The example of a training checklist in Figure 4.4 lists various technical skills assistants and technicians routinely need to be able to complete. This type of checklist is particularly useful because it can track not only the completion of a job task but also the level of proficiency. Notice the checklist includes multiple lines by each item signifying the skill must be performed multiple times. Supervisors can write their initials when an employee successfully completes a specific skill such as setting an intravenous catheter. This ensures team members truly have mastered the knowledge and skills they need to excel rather than just performing a skill once.

There are many training tools that help team members learn. Bear in mind training tools work much better when used actively vs. passively. Telling a team member, for example, that they can read training guides to learn the practice management software is not likely to be nearly as effective as allotting 30-minute sessions for a new hire to read the guide and then practice what they learned.

Here are examples of tools and resources to use for training:

- Articles
- Books
- Podcasts
- Written training guides (subject matter notes, instructions, outlines, protocols)
- Online training: webinars, videos and courses on virtual training platforms, websites
- Journal clubs
- In-house seminars presented by practice leaders
- Lunch n Learns from industry partners
- In person seminars and workshops

If you've ever had a team member that was a slow learner, continued to make mistakes or avoided completing certain job duties, the problem might be they didn't receive adequate training or never achieved a level of expertise needed to do their job well. Here are resources and tools you can use to evaluate an employee's retention and ability:

- Quizzes
- Q&A with trainers or mentors
- Hands-on assignments to assess competency
- Online assessments included with virtual training courses

Learning Styles

People have different preferred learning styles so consider whether your training programs help facilitate learning for everyone. Three of the most common learning styles are based on main sensory receivers: visual, auditory, and kinesthetic (VAK). The concept is that visual learners prefer to view diagrams, charts, and pictures as a major part of learning, auditory learners like to hear the presenter and kinesthetic learners prefer hands-on training or interactive participation.[4] Many educators believe people learn best when taught according to their identified learning style, however, research indicates there may not be scientific evidence to support this premise. Studies have shown that while people may self-identify as a specific type of learner, this doesn't mean they have more ability to learn with that specific style of instruction.[5]

It does make sense to inquire whether team members have preferences on how they like to learn because this can help to tailor training for individuals. Some employees may learn better with self-study while others may prefer to learn with a group. But using a combination of education methods will likely maximize learning and lead to the best outcomes for the practice. Some skills, for example, need to be taught with hands-on instruction. No amount of reading can replace the physical process of learning how to draw blood from patients. To gain competence, team members need to practice venipuncture. On the other hand, studying written handouts will definitely help augment the learning process of hearing a co-worker verbally explain vaccine schedules.

Don't forget pet owners have different styles of learning as well so it's a good idea for the team to discuss effective ways to educate clients. When teams understand the common ways people like to learn they may be more likely to use a variety of communications and educational tools to enhance the overall learning experience for clients. This helps to gain greater client compliance because pet owners are more likely to agree to treatment recommendations if they fully appreciate the need for a service and fully understand the value of the service. Client education and compliance are covered in detail in Chapter 10 on Marketing and Client Communications.

LEADERSHIP TRAINING FOR MIDDLE MANAGERS

Often businesses promote team members from within the organization to middle management positions. Practices may promote a veterinary technician or assistant to be the technician supervisor, or a team lead in the department. Likewise, the practice might promote a client service representative to office manager or team lead at the front desk. Other examples of job positions in the hospital with some managerial duties include roles such as senior technician, training manager, client services coordinator, referring veterinarian liaison, inventory manager, operations manager, and project team leader.

Some employees receive promotions because they asked for more responsibility but in many instances, practices promote team members who demonstrate high levels of proficiency, a strong work ethic, or have years of experience in their current job. But just because someone excels in their current job role doesn't mean they'll be successful in a management position. Unwittingly, practice owners and practice managers may set team members up to fail if they don't provide middle managers with appropriate management and leadership training. Without the proper tools and resources they need to be effective in their new role, middle managers may experience frustration, burn-out, and problems with job performance. Moreover, without proper guidance and training, they aren't as likely to succeed with their efforts related to team development.

Ideally, the first step before promoting someone into a managerial role is to define the requisite skills, talents, and job performance for the position. This helps to avoid giving a promotion to a team member simply because they have tenure, want the job, or have excellent technical skills. Anyone in a management or team leader role needs to possess positive leadership skills, a desire to learn, and an ability to embrace change. Prior to offering a new position, consider whether an employee has shown an aptitude for leadership and whether they're likely to be open to receiving feedback on how they can improve. Remember that a middle manager needs to be a positive role model and demonstrate behavior aligned with the practice's core values. This means always being on-time to work, avoiding gossip, eliminating any favoritism towards team members, and being able to provide objective feedback to co-workers who may be their friends.

An often-overlooked aspect of effectively transitioning a team member into a managerial role is to clearly define their new job duties and expectations. Simply agreeing that a team lead or supervisor will start overseeing workflow doesn't provide enough clarity about the new job responsibilities. Middle managers need a job description that outlines details about their new job roles and expectations. For example, will they now be actively involved in employee recruitment activities such as reviewing resumes and setting up interviews? Are they responsible for implementing training programs and meeting with team members to discuss their development? What added job duties will they have such as equipment maintenance or staff scheduling? Will they be expected to work a different work schedule at times or be available for overtime? Will they need to learn new skills, attend continuing education sessions and/or be present at manager meetings? If your practice didn't define these aspects of the job role when a team member became a middle manager, remember that it's never too late to gain clarity and discuss job performance expectations.

Middle managers also need to understand the level of authority and autonomy that goes along with their position. A team leader, for example, generally doesn't have the same level of authority as a technician supervisor. The team leader may handle making daily job assignments, directing workflow, and checking to make sure everyone completes all their work by the end of the shift. But they may not be responsible for discussing job performance problems with their co-workers. A supervisor, on the other hand, may be responsible for addressing lack of accountability, giving negative feedback, and making hiring decisions. The entire team also needs to understand the level of responsibility of middle managers, so they know who they report to and the flow of communication in the hospital. For example, team members need to know if they are supposed to bring concerns to the attention of a middle manager, the practice manager, or the business owner.

Middle managers may face a number of different challenges. They may have to balance completing their current job duties and new management duties. Younger team members may be in a position of supervising co-workers who are older, have been with the practice longer, or are their friends. An experienced veterinary assistant might be a supervisor for credentialed technicians. And employees promoted into middle management positions without direct supervisory responsibilities may still need to gain cooperation from their co-workers. These situations can be tricky to navigate. Any team member in a middle management role needs to know how to influence their teammates and motivate them to work together to achieve hospital goals.

As members of the practice's leadership team, middle managers need education and coaching in the following areas:

- Being a positive role model
- How to manage by core values
- Effective time management

- How to manage up
- Communication skills to build trust
- Giving positive and negative feedback
- How to promote teamwork and accountability with their peers
- How to set boundaries and clarify expectations
- Conflict resolution skills
- Self-leadership
- Work-life balance and self-care

Other chapters of this book provide instruction and guidance in the above topic areas. Note that Chapter 6 on Employee Retention covers how to implement development plans for team members so they can continue to learn and grow in their jobs. Development plans for middle managers should include a separate section that outlines goals for leadership development. You want a technician supervisor, for example, to gain new technical skills but you also want them to gain expertise as a manager. The areas of focus for a middle manager's leadership development will depend on their current skill set, level of experience, and individual needs. The development plan should include specific action steps to attain goals, what resources to access, and a timeline to accomplish the goals. Resources may include books, management articles, Ted talks, podcasts, webinars, and continuing education conferences.

At a minimum, middle managers need to receive on-going guidance from their direct supervisor. They can also benefit immensely from being coached and mentored by another member of the team with more experience. Mentors may be practice managers, associate veterinarians, practice owners, regional managers or another senior member of the leadership team. Even if you don't have a formal mentorship program, make sure middle managers know who to talk to about their challenges and development progress. In addition to traditional mentorship, many companies now implement reverse-mentoring programs. With these programs, someone with less experience or tenure may mentor another co-worker or even their manager. For example, a young employee who is particularly knowledgeable about social media and technology may mentor the technician supervisor on how to recruit younger generations or a team member who is African American may mentor their manager on diversity topics.[6]

SUMMARY

The goal of creating and implementing a comprehensive training program for the entire team may seem overwhelming at the beginning of the project. It's easy to lose focus on employee training since managers have so many other competing projects and job duties. But practices that make training a priority reap the benefits of increased employee satisfaction, retention, and productivity. Training programs are an integral part of employee development which is a topic included in Chapter 6 on Employee Retention. And of course, practices are more successful when employees gain advanced knowledge and skills that improve patient care and client communications.

As you learned in Chapter 1, the secret to achieving a large goal is to break it down into smaller, reasonable goals you can accomplish in a shorter time period. Regardless of whether you have a detailed training program or are just starting this project, look at the big picture by creating an outline of the practice's desired training program. This makes it easier to see what training programs you need to develop, what tools and resources you might need and the direction to take to prioritize action steps to reach goals. For example, you may have excellent training in place for veterinary assistants and technicians but not for client service representatives. Maybe you now recognize you need better orientation and on-boarding programs for new hires.

Since employee training is vital to the success of your business, strive to have an organized program that employees can consistently access to learn and become more proficient in their jobs. Don't forget the necessity of delegating part of the workload to multiple team members; managers simply cannot do it all when it comes to training. Likewise, don't forget to evaluate the practice's training program on an annual basis at a minimum. This helps ensure all written documents and supporting resources are sufficient and accurate as well as uncover if there are new training needs. The annual review should also assess whether current training programs are effective at achieving the desired outcome of efficiently improving the skills, knowledge, and abilities of all team members.

CHAPTER 5

Enhancing and Evaluating Job Performance

Whether an employee is going through the on-boarding process during their first year of employment or has worked at the practice for many years, they need to be given every opportunity to enhance their job performance. Likewise, team members need regular feedback and job performance evaluations, so they know if they're meeting job expectations and if not, what they need to do to improve. Helping people reach higher levels of job performance benefits the practice by increasing employee job satisfaction, productivity, and retention.

The last thing any manager wants is to recruit and train a team member only to have them experience trouble performing their job duties or quit. In this chapter, you will learn ways to try to ensure that doesn't happen. Each section explains fundamental elements of human resource management and team development. Sometimes, problems with job performance are a result of skipping the employee communications outlined in this chapter. Therefore, you may want to refer to the information presented here anytime a team member is struggling in their job.

MANAGING BY CORE VALUES

In Chapter 2 on Enhancing Culture, you learned how to define your organization's core values and how they are the roadmap for employee behavior. You discovered the importance of connecting all areas of management and team communications to the core values. Now, we look further at how to manage by core values because this process supports guiding team members to higher levels of job performance. In the rest of this chapter, you will see how to reference core values when talking to employees, so they better understand their purpose at work and how their job performance fits into the mission and vision of the practice.

To effectively manage by core values, the values must be a focus for the team, so they become part of the culture. It isn't enough to include core values in the employee policy manual or post them on a plaque in the hospital. While these may be good reminders, the presence of core values in a handbook or on a wall doesn't mean everyone understands them or lives them. Team members need clarity about how their job performance must align with the values of the business. Therefore, it's best to talk about the practice's core values when delegating job duties, giving feedback, holding accountability meetings, conducting job performance reviews, and during disciplinary meetings.

When discussing whether an employee's job performance aligns with core values, help people understand the outcomes of their actions. This is especially true if someone doesn't think what they did (or didn't do) is a big deal. Perhaps, you need to talk to a team member about their chronic tardiness. If they're only 10-15 minutes late, they may not see this as a major problem. But as the manager, you know the negative effects tardiness can have on patient care, client care, teamwork, productivity, and morale. If one of the practice's core values is respect, you might explain that showing up late demonstrates a lack of respect for co-workers and clients. Moreover, point out to this employee specifically how tardiness has adverse effects on the entire team as well as pet owners.

Another powerful way to weave core values into team communications is to celebrate behaviors aligned with core values by sharing success stories. This can be done during monthly meetings or weekly standing meetings by having team members share experiences about something they did or observed that had a positive effect on patients, clients, co-workers, or the community that upholds the core values. Here's an example: "I saw Sally assist Mrs. Jones with her children. Her child, Lucas, was frustrated and close to having a temper tantrum. Sally took him on a tour of the hospital and showed him some kittens that were boarding. He returned to his mom all smiles. Her actions support our core value of compassion." Notice this is a feel-good story everyone can enjoy and that it includes specific details about actions Sally took to show her compassion.

It's worth noting that citing the practice's core values when talking to employees about their job performance may sound awkward or even phony if you are just starting to manage by core values. The first key to your success is to strive to sound conversational. You don't have to rehearse perfect sounding sentences. The second key is to avoid joking or using humor because this detracts from the seriousness of creating a values-based culture. And third, consistency is critical. Stay the course; reference core values every opportunity that comes your way and you will be able to build a positive culture of high performers. Creating a values-based organization takes time. You know you're making progress when employees who aren't members of the leadership team talk about the core values without being prompted.

Bear in mind managing by core values only works well if you and the rest of the practice leaders model behaviors that support the core values. Otherwise, what you say may sound disingenuous or fall on deaf ears, and team members just see the core values as words on paper. Let's say, for example, your practice has a core value of "Innovation: We will strive to continuously improve patient care and use state-of-the-art technology to provide the most successful treatment." You could appropriately refer to this core value when talking to a team member about how they need to be more committed to learning how to use a new piece of equipment. But what if this employee presented their ideas on how to improve post-surgical patient care three weeks prior and you were distracted, didn't appear interested in their proposed protocol change, or didn't follow-through? In instances such as this, team members may perceive the leadership team isn't living the core values of the business.

EFFECTIVE DELEGATION

In the workplace, to delegate means to direct or instruct someone to complete a job task. To delegate also means to allocate responsibility to employees to accomplish their assigned job duties. Aside from basic job duties outlined in their job description, managers may delegate additional job tasks or projects to team members. Delegation is an effective way for managers to gain assistance to complete projects and achieve hospital goals. By delegating certain job duties, managers can focus more on essential work only they are qualified to do such as financial management. The value of delegation for the team includes increased efficiency, more creativity, better decision-making, and providing employees opportunities for growth.

Problems may arise if managers don't see the connection between delegation and enhancing the job performance of team members. Specifically, managers may not understand that a failure to delegate can limit an employee's job performance because they aren't even given a chance to excel. An unwillingness to delegate generally occurs for two reasons which involve short-sighted thinking. First, managers may feel they don't have time to delegate and think, "It's just faster if I do this myself." Second, managers sometimes assess they're the only one who can correctly complete job tasks or projects. While this may legitimately be true, it's worth taking the time to train an employee so they can assume more job responsibilities moving forward.

Defining Job Duties, Roles, and Expectations

Essentially, delegation begins during the employee on-boarding process as new hires learn and assume responsibility to complete their job duties. Delegation sounds simple enough. So, why don't all team members consistently finish their work? Why don't all employees have the same level of job performance? And when given additional job assignments, why doesn't everyone complete them on time? The answer to these questions often relates to how managers communicate with employees when delegating job duties. Simply asking or instructing an employee to do a job task, doesn't always yield positive results. This is because for delegation to work well, managers need to ensure team members understand how to achieve desired outcomes.[1]

At a minimum, employees need clearly defined job descriptions that include job expectations, so they understand their job requirements and responsibilities. The purpose of job descriptions is to establish the foundation for desired job performance. But job descriptions alone don't result in successful outcomes for delegation. To achieve desired outcomes, you need to effectively communicate with team members when delegating job duties. Using the following five-step process is an excellent way to set employees up for success when delegating work. (See Figure 5.1 for a summary of an effective delegation process.)

1. Establish the value of job assignments.

Discuss the value of job tasks to avoid having employees feel like you're dumping work on them. If you need to complete inventory counts, for example, it makes sense to have several people help with this project. But team members won't be excited about counting pills so let them know how accurate inventory counts relate to effective inventory management which in turns helps the practice save money.

2. Establish job expectations.

When assigning job tasks, clarify how and when employees need to complete work. This is important whether you ask a team member to mop a floor, take radiographs, or start a senior care program. Establishing specific job expectations helps to avoid misunderstandings and communication breakdowns. Let's say the responsibility of basic patient care for pets in an isolation ward is delegated to a relatively new veterinary assistant. It would be important to inform this employee if they were to use bleach when cleaning rather than assuming they know which product to use. Likewise, a veterinary technician tasked with setting up a senior care program needs direction and guidance, so they don't waste time working on a project that isn't what the leadership team wants.

3. Set priorities.

Team members need to understand their priorities especially if they must juggle multiple job duties. A client service representative responsible for handling prescription refills, completing audits for missed charges, and preparing puppy/kitten kits may not

Table 5.1: Effective Delegation Process

Steps	Description
Establish the Value of Job Assignments	State benefits related to job duties and link to core values. Example: "Calling pet owners to alert them about overdue preventive care for their pet helps them remember to schedule appointments and is consistent with our core value of patient advocacy."
Establish Job Expectations	Provide guidance about how job duties must be completed. State any relevant details related to job tasks.
Set Priorities	Communicate the order of priority and which job tasks are to be completed first.
Check for Understanding	Ask team members whether they have questions about assigned job duties. Use an open-ended question such as "What questions do you have?"
Agree on Deadlines	Ask team members how much time they need to complete assignments. Agree upon specific deadlines.

conclude that filling prescription requests as soon as it is received is more important than the other two competing job tasks. Therefore, it's critical to prioritize job duties when delegating additional assignments. Similarly, a technician or assistant asked to do bloodwork, set an IV catheter, and do radiographs on three different patients, needs to know if the veterinarian wants treatments for one of these pet's to be a priority.

4. Check for understanding.

While it may seem unnecessary, verify that team members understand what they're supposed to do and how they're expected to do it. You can do this by asking employees an open-ended question to check for their understanding. You might ask "What questions do you have about this assignment?" or "Tell me what concerns you have about completing this project." Notice, that because these are open-end questions, someone can't reasonably just answer "yes" or "no." Instead, they will likely indicate comprehension with a response such as "I got it" or they may ask for clarification about your expectations. This is also the time when employees tend to indicate if they aren't on-board with the assignment or don't buy-in to the value of the assignment which gives you a chance to address their concerns.

5. Agree on deadlines.

This is a critical part of the communication process. Team members inherently understand deadlines related to the daily workload. But when job duties don't have to be completed right away, clarify the deadline. This is especially true when the employee has a history of lack of accountability. If the timeline is flexible, ask the team member what they think is a reasonable deadline. This helps to gain buy-in because they set the deadline. If they offer a timeline that is different than yours, you can negotiate an agreed upon deadline. Remember, team members may need to have time allocated for them to complete requested job tasks that are outside the scope of the regular job duties. Be sure to specify dates and times, not general timelines. For example, rather than saying "in a few days" set a deadline of "Friday at 5pm."

Oversight Vs. Micro-Management

Part of being a good manager involves overseeing the job performance of the team. In fact, just because you delegate job duties to employees doesn't mean you give up your accountability to the practice owners. Managers are responsible for making sure employees successfully complete work that is delegated. Whether your supervisor is the practice owner, a hospital administrator, a medical director, or a regional manager, they won't be happy if they ask about an unfinished project and you respond by saying "Oh, I delegated that to Jill. I assumed she finished it."

Following up with employees is especially important when giving responsibility to new employees or when making assignments for the first time. Once team members have a proven job performance, you won't need to check in as frequently. Of course, checking in with employees to see how they're doing, whether they have questions about assignments, and to provide feedback if appropriate is not the same as micromanagement. Oversight and striving to help team members enhance their job performance is distinctly different than micromanaging employees.

So, what exactly is micromanagement? How do you know if you're a micromanager? What do you need to do to change if you realize you tend to micromanage? The answer to these questions lies in understanding micromanagement. Honestly assessing how you interact with employees and how you delegate is critical. Asking team members how they feel about your management style is also helpful. Even if they don't use the word micromanagement, you may hear feedback that suggests you tend to be a micromanager. (For characteristics of micromanagers, see textbox, "Signs That You May Be a Micromanager.")

Perhaps the best word to think of in association with micromanagement is control. When people micromanage, they may be reluctant to delegate because they don't trust employees to do a good job. Micromanagers tend to hover or constantly check up on employees to confirm they're doing their jobs. Another hallmark of micromanagers is they focus on every small detail of how employees perform their job even when it isn't important. An example would be assigning someone to create a bulletin board or display focused on the importance of heartworm prevention and then re-arranging the display once they finish the project. This type of micromanagement shuts down creativity and decreases employee motivation. Another example of control happens when managers tell employees every decision must be approved by them. This stifles initiative, decreases efficiency, and lowers morale.

Not only does micromanagement have damaging effects on employees' job performance, it also hinders the success of managers. Failure to effectively delegate means being stuck doing more work. Sometimes managers confuse trying to hold employees accountable with micromanagement. Their efforts to move team members to a higher level of job performance have the opposite effect. As you will read shortly, enhancing accountability is achieved with specific communications, not by asserting control over employees.

If you believe you may be guilty of micromanagement, there are strategies you can use to change. One is to give up on perfection and let go of details that don't matter. Of course, medical protocols need to be followed and data must be entered correctly into the practice management software. But does it matter how the break room is organized? Do you need to approve every social media post once team members know their guidelines? Do you need to voice how you would have taken a different approach to the kennel staff schedule as long as all the shifts are covered? Hopefully, you answered no to these questions.

> **Signs You May Be a Micromanager**
>
> - You focus on exactly how a job task must be done rather than the desired results.
> - You feel like no-one on the team pays enough attention to details like you would.
> - You frequently find yourself correcting work assignments.
> - You're always watching to make sure everyone is working.
> - You insist team members always get approval before acting.
> - Your boss asks why you're completing job tasks someone else could do.
> - You insist on being a part of every meeting held by other team members-e.g., your project team or training team.
> - You hear team members express that nothing they do is good enough. They feel you're never satisfied with their work.

Another strategy is to discuss relevant details of delegated job duties when you make assignments. This doesn't mean telling employees exactly how to complete their work but rather ensures you provide clear direction on how to approach the project when appropriate and the desired outcome. This is also an ideal time to ask employees to convey their ideas about how they will approach a project or complete assigned work. Creating dialogue with employees gives you an opportunity to ask questions and offer feedback if appropriate.

FEEDBACK

Giving feedback is unquestionably a primary way to enhance job performance. Through the process of feedback, people learn whether they're doing a good job or need to make improvements. Effective feedback helps keep team members on track to meet or exceed expectations when fulfilling their job assignments. Without feedback, team members are left to make their own assessments which may or not be accurate and aligned with what management thinks. Unfortunately, sometimes employees only hear about their job performance during formal reviews or when they do something wrong. An analysis by Gallup revealed 47% of employees said they only received feedback "a few times a

Enhancing and Evaluating Job Performance

year or less."[2] (See Figure 5.3: How Often Employees Say They Receive Feedback From Their Managers.)

When managers provide consistent feedback, they reinforce the desired behavior from team members and are more likely to ensure employees understand work assignments. It's relevant to note that an effective feedback process includes asking for feedback from employees, not just giving them feedback. Here are good questions to ask to solicit employee feedback:

- How are you doing in your job?
- Do you have everything you need to do your job?
- What do you need from me to do your job better?
- What challenges do you need help with?
- What ideas do you have related to your job roles?

Figure 5.1: How Often Employees Say They Receive Feedback From Their Managers

How often do you receive feedback from your manager?

- Once a year or less: 19%
- A few times a year: 28%
- A few times a month: 27%
- A few times a week: 19%
- Daily: 7%

Percentage of respondents who have received feedback from their managers, by frequency

Source: Adapted from "The Ultimate Guide to Micromanagers: Signs, Causes, Solutions" by Ben Wigert and Ryan Pendell, https://www.gallup.com/workplace/315530/ultimate-guide-micromanagers-signs-causes-solutions.aspx, July 17, 2020.

How To Give Meaningful Feedback

There is an art to giving effective feedback. (See Table 5.2: Characteristics of Effective vs. Ineffective Feedback.) The last thing you want is to give feedback that inadvertently decreases motivation or morale. To give meaningful feedback, the first key is to genuinely want to help team members succeed and to give them every opportunity to enhance their job performance. Even if there are aspects of an employee's personality, behavior, or job performance that are vexing at times, managers must treat everyone fairly and include them in the feedback process.

Another key to make feedback more relevant and powerful, is to tell employees how their actions either are or are not aligned with the core values of the practice. When giving positive feedback, you might say "Your kind words and compassion towards Mrs. Jones were evident and your actions are aligned with our core value of providing exemplary service. Thank you for your dedication to our clients." If you were giving negative feedback to a team member who didn't complete patient treatments appropriately, you might say "Your failure to give Rocky his medication could be detrimental to his well-being. Your actions don't support our core value of providing high quality patient care. I need you to give all patient treatments as directed moving forward."

Be aware of appropriate times and places to give feedback. It's fine to give an employee positive feedback where co-workers may hear what you say. But when the need arises to give feedback about inconsistent job performance or failure to complete job tasks, set up a private meeting with employees. Feedback does need to be timely to have the most benefit so strive to offer feedback as quickly as possible after observed behavior. Memories tend to fade so delayed feedback may not be accurate or seem as valuable to someone. Moreover, it's easy to forget about giving feedback or decide that it isn't that important if you wait too long. Always try to give feedback the same day as observed behavior if possible and if not, then the next time the employee works.

Another important aspect of feedback is for it to be specific. Giving details about *how* job duties are performed is more meaningful than general comments. Instead of saying "Thanks for doing a good job" it's better to say "Thank you for staying an hour late on Tuesday. I know that was incredibly helpful to Dr. Smith and beneficial to our patients." Specific feedback lets team members know what behavior they should continue and what behavior is unacceptable. Like it or not, employees don't all have the same definition of what is an "exceptional, good or poor" job performance, what is "on-time" or what is "friendly client service."

Always focus feedback on the behavior not the person. This means feedback needs to concentrate on the observed behavior of the team member not on something you can't unequivocally know such as their attitude or intention. While you can't measure, quantify, or see an employee's attitude or intention, you can observe their behavior and actions. Informing an employee that they need to have a better attitude or be nicer to pet owners may be confusing or debatable if the team member doesn't understand why there's a problem with their actions. In these instances, telling someone "You weren't nice to Mrs. Jones" doesn't help enhance job performance. But saying "I noticed you raised your voice with Mrs. Jones and cut her off when she was talking" identifies the unacceptable behavior. Feedback that references specific behavior and actions helps employees better understand how they need to perform their job.

Table 5.2: Characteristics of Effective vs. Ineffective Feedback

Characteristic	Effective	Ineffective
Timely	Given within hours or the same day	Given weeks later or never
Specific	"Your efforts to increase dental care compliance by communicating value to clients and forward booking have helped us increase compliance by 15%."	"Great job everyone."
Focus on core values	"When you show up late you demonstrate a lack of respect for your co-workers."	"You're late and I want you to be on time."
Focus on observed behavior, not the person	"I observed you stalking off and muttering under your breath about how busy you are when Jill asked for help."	"You never want to help your teammates."
Consistent	Given daily or weekly	Only given when someone does something wrong or during reviews

Giving Negative Feedback Positively

Practice owners and managers often dread giving negative feedback because it makes them uncomfortable or they're afraid it's discouraging and demotivating. They may procrastinate confronting team members about their inferior job performance or use what has been called "the sandwich approach" when giving feedback. With this technique, negative feedback is voiced between two positive pieces of feedback. Managers might do this because they think it softens the blow for employees or because it makes it easier for them to deliver uncomfortable feedback. People who use this method of feedback think they're being fair and kind but in actuality, giving feedback this way can hinder rather than enhance job performance. Combining positive feedback with negative feedback is confusing. A team member may leave the meeting thinking, "I guess I'm doing pretty well." Additionally, the value of the positive feedback may be diminished if employees think it isn't sincere.[3]

Note that negative feedback actually helps people understand what they need to do to improve their job performance because it is *informative*. If negative feedback is disguised or unclear due to your attempts to sugarcoat the message, you aren't doing your employees any favors. Consider that according to Gallup research, only 26% of employees strongly agree that the feedback they receive helps them perform better.[4] So rather than avoid negative feedback, it's vital to learn how to communicate negative feedback in a positive way that is beneficial for employees.

One way to give negative feedback effectively is to be specific about what aspect of the job performance needs correction so people don't overgeneralize that they're a bad employee. This is particularly important when talking to new hires, inexperienced employees, or people you perceive to have low self-esteem because they're more likely to take negative feedback personally.[5] Let's say you want to convey negative feedback to a client service representative new to veterinary medicine about their communication skills. Specify which skills they need to work on and why. Rather than saying "Emily, your communication is abrupt and lacks warmth", you would say "Emily, it's critical to show our clients how much we care about them and their pets. To do this, I'd like you to start practicing these two skills with every client. I want you to smile at every client and make meaningful eye contact while talking to them. This will help you show clients that you're interested and care about them."

When giving negative feedback, it's tempting to use phrases such as "I know you tried" or "I know interacting with difficult clients isn't your strength." Similar to the sandwich technique, the problem with this feedback is that it lets someone off the hook for accepting responsibility for their unacceptable job performance. Additionally, this type of feedback may suggest that you don't think they can excel or worse yet leave employees feeling depressed.[6] To avoid this scenario, give direct negative feedback while emphasizing you're confident the employee can successfully improve. You might say, "I know Mrs. Young can be difficult to communicate with. I didn't see you engage with her the same way you do with other clients. We've discussed ways to handle difficult clients. Let's discuss your challenges and come up with a plan for you to re-commit to using specific communication skills with clients like Mrs. Young."

Another word to avoid when giving feedback is the word *but* because it minimizes or negates whatever was said before the word but. Here's an example: "John, you did an excellent job placing that IV catheter, but you didn't clip the hair in a wide enough margin before setting the catheter." If John had successfully placed an IV catheter for the first time in a breed such as a dachshund, the negative feedback following the positive takes away from the praise. Rather than saying *but*, use the word *and* instead or simply separate the negative and positive feedback completely into different sentences as follows: "John, you did an excellent job placing that IV catheter. It can be difficult to place catheters in dachshunds. You started the catheter in the right place, and it looks great. I noticed you didn't follow the proper medical protocol when clipping Gretchen's hair. What questions do you have about how to do this properly next time?" Notice that in the second example, there is no admonishment telling John to follow the protocol but instead, you seek to uncover if he doesn't understand the protocol. This helps to determine if John needs further training and helps gain buy-in regarding the importance of medical standards.

ACCOUNTABILITY

Accountability refers to people taking responsibility for their actions as well as taking initiative and ownership of the results of one's actions. Lack of accountability in the workplace refers to a failure to do job duties properly and/or an unwillingness to accept responsibility for successfully completing job tasks. Employees may demonstrate a lack of accountability related to just one job duty or multiple aspects of their job. They may have an occasional lapse in job performance or demonstrate a consistent lack of accountability. Team members who lack accountability often give excuses for their behavior or verbalize thoughts such as "It's good enough" Iit's not my job", "I didn't have time", "I didn't know", or "I just work here."

Individual and team job performance suffers when employees aren't accountable. When managers fail to address problems with accountability, multiple problems arise. The practice may experience decreased efficiency and productivity as well as ineffective teamwork and low morale. Additionally, lack of accountability may negatively affect patient care and client service. Therefore, it's imperative to address lack of accountability quickly.

Identifying Causes of Lack of Accountability

Since there are different underlying causes for lack of accountability, try to identify which factors are relevant so you can put in place appropriate strategies to improve the team member's job performance. If an employee isn't accountable due to a lack of integrity, for example, they may need to be terminated. On the other hand, if someone lacks accountability because they haven't received sufficient training, you can implement steps to help them attain the knowledge and skills they need to excel. Lack of training is one of the most common causes for a lack of accountability. (See Figure 5.3 for the primary causes and characteristics of lack of accountability.)

Table 5.3: Lack of Accountability: Causes and Characteristics

Causes of Lack of Accountability	Characteristics
A lack of integrity	Team members who violate the code of conduct, lack a moral compass Examples: lying, stealing, dishonesty, lack of respect, insubordination
Ineffective training	Often an overlooked problem Look for evidence that an employee wants to do a good job but lacks knowledge or skills
Unclear job expectations	Job performance suffers because employees' roles and responsibilities are unclear Look for valid feedback that team members didn't know they were responsible for a job duty
Lack of clarity about policies or protocols	Confusion about policies and protocols Practice lacks written protocols and updated policies Look for evidence that multiple employees don't know what to do
Outside influences	Team members may have personal problems or challenges that negatively affect job performance Examples: illness, relationship discord, substance abuse, childcare or caregiver challenges
Poor job fit	Employees who don't excel despite training, feedback, and development opportunities
Suboptimal motivation	Employees who are disillusioned, disengaged, or disgruntled
Lack of consequences	Unacceptable job performance continues due to a lack of consequences for poor behavior

When assessing lack of accountability, evaluate whether the problem rests with just one or two employees or is a problem with the entire team. When multiple team members lack accountability, the underlying issue usually involves insufficient training or a lack of clarity regarding job expectations, procedures, or protocols. Regardless of the reasons for employees being unaccountable, it's the manager's responsibility to talk to them about the problem and what corrective action they need to take.

Holding Effective Accountability Meetings

When employees lack accountability, this doesn't necessarily mean they need to be formally disciplined. Perhaps an experienced team member makes a significant mistake or acts in a way that is out of character. Maybe a new hire doesn't finish their assigned job duties. Or perhaps you notice an employee has been tardy multiple times in the last month. These circumstances warrant meeting with a team member to identify factors related to their poor job performance and agree on a plan to meet job expectations. But they don't necessarily call for disciplinary action.

If you prepare for employee accountability meetings and follow a defined process, you'll be more likely to achieve positive outcomes. To facilitate a successful meeting, it's always best to assume a team member has the best intentions because this helps set an optimistic tone. People usually want to do a good job and appreciate the opportunity to discuss how they can enhance their performance. It's also important to monitor your emotions and avoid scheduling meetings if you're angry or upset. Take a few hours or a day if necessary so you can maintain your composure during the meeting. Lastly, organize an agenda so you're ready to present specific, factual information to employees about observed behavior and use the communication techniques outlined above to give effective feedback. (See Table 5.4 for a communication process you can use for accountability meetings.)

As a manager, you want to create a culture of accountability but also consider whether you can hold someone accountable. You've undoubtedly heard the phrase "You need to hold your employees accountable." Is that possible? What is your role in making that a reality? While it's true managers are responsible for the oversight of team performance, you can't control what action employees take to improve or whether they succeed. Cy Wakeman, founder of Reality-Based Leadership, is a drama researcher who points out that accountability is a mindset and people have a choice. She recommends managers avoid trying to assert power over people but instead promote and insist upon personal accountability.[7] In Chapter 7 on Communications Challenges and Solutions you'll learn more about the best ways to motivate employees and encourage self-leadership.

Table 5.4: Communication Process for Accountability Meetings

Steps	Description
Step 1: Clearly and succinctly state the purpose of the meeting.	Explain gaps in job expectations and actual job performance.
	Focus on facts and observed behavior; give specific examples of lack of accountability.
	Convey goal to create a mutually desirable outcome of improved job performance and retention of a valued team member.
Step 2: Focus on core values.	Clearly communicate behaviors that violate core values.
	Anchor team members to behaviors aligned with core values.
Step 3. Solicit feedback from team members to determine relevant factors related to accountability.	Ask "What is your view?"
	Ask "Tell me your thoughts."
Step 4. Actively listen; determine if employees have valid feedback or unmet needs vs excuses and justifications for behavior.	Look for barriers or competing priorities.
	Listen for evidence of lack of training or clarity about protocols.
	Determine if problems with job performance appears to be suboptimal motivation or lack of ability (it could be both).
Step 5. Avoid trying to fix the problem; Ask employees for their solutions and ideas.	Ask "How can you solve this problem?"
	Ask "What assistance do you need to do your job better?"
Step 6. Establish clear consequences for poor performance or bad behavior.	Convey any negative impact on patients, the team, clients, and the practice.
	Explain the risk to job security, possible initiation of progressive discipline.

LEGAL ISSUES

To avoid discrimination claims and lawsuits, all practices need to have an employee handbook that includes statements regarding the company's compliance with all employment laws, a code of conduct, an anti-harassment policy, an outline of disciplinary procedures, a disclaimer that nothing in the handbook creates a contract for employment, and an acknowledgement of receipt page for employees to sign. In addition, employers must clearly understand their responsibilities related to employee job performance reviews, discipline, and termination to avoid discrimination charges or lawsuits. This is a critical component of human resources compliance which is the process of defining your policies and procedures to ensure the practice complies with all applicable laws related to employees in the workplace.[8] Compliance with all federal, state, and local laws is imperative as the effects of discrimination claims or illegal actions can be costly and damaging to the practice culture. In addition to being educated, it's prudent for managers to utilize outside companies that provide assistance on compliance issues and an attorney with expertise in employment law.

Avoiding Discrimination

Take care to avoid discrimination when conducting job performance reviews, during disciplinary procedures, and when firing employees. Make sure all management actions don't discriminate against team members on the basis of age, (40 or older), sex (including pregnancy, sexual orientation, and gender identity), race, religion, color, national origin, disability, or genetic information (including family medical history). It's essential to keep documentation for all employee meetings since they may later be needed to defend the business if a complaint is filed.[9]

You may not think about the possibility of discrimination occurring when conducting job performance reviews but there are several common mistakes employers make that you want to be sure to avoid. Perhaps the most obvious one is to side-step referring to an employee's pregnancy or other medical condition during the review. A simple statement such as "I know you must be tired due to your pregnancy" or "I know it can be difficult dealing with chronic illness" may seem innocuous but could be perceived negatively by an employee and lead to a discrimination claim.

Another common mistake is to make unclear statements about a team member that could be misinterpreted. Telling someone, for example, that they don't have a good work ethic or aren't a good team player are vague labels that should be avoided. These references focus on the person rather than their behavior and don't specify what job duties aren't being accomplished. Equally problematic is giving an employee praise and indicating they have a future with the company despite their poor job performance. An employee who is disciplined or terminated at a later date could use these types of written or expressed statements as evidence you have discriminated against them.[10]

Practices must also avoid discrimination by making sure there is a consistent review process for all team members. Review procedures need to be the completed the same way for everyone. It's important to schedule reviews on the same timetable for the entire team rather than preferentially holding reviews for certain employees. And consistent protocols need to be followed. For example, if associate veterinarians or middle managers are part of the review process, they need to review all team members they work with not just a select few. Use the same or similar review forms for all departments that apply the same standards for all team members. Review forms for veterinary technicians and assistants, for example, should specify the level of proficiency that must be demonstrated to achieve higher ratings for specific technical skills such as setting intravenous catheters. This helps ensure practice leaders who review employees use objective criteria and rate employees consistently. Remember that skills listed do need to be consistent with what is allowed by the state's veterinary medicine practice act.

As with reviews, employee discipline must be consistent and fair. Discipline given to one team member for inferior job performance or misconduct must be the same for another team member who has similar problems or commits the same infraction. Otherwise, the business is subject to discrimination claims. Consider, for example, if a manager showed favoritism towards a young employee who is chronically tardy by allowing the behavior to continue but initiated disciplinary procedures against an older employee. Consider if an African American team member was disciplined for poor job performance, but their White co-worker made the same mistakes and wasn't disciplined. In both these instances, employees may have valid claims for discrimination.

Documentation

The importance of documenting all employee communications related to job performance cannot be overstated. Having a written record of how well employees meet job expectations helps managers keep track of job performance and fairly administer discipline. Documentation, or lack thereof, could also be directly related to whether the company can protect itself against discrimination claims and successfully win lawsuits. With proper documentation, employers can show employees were disciplined or let go for valid reasons not because of illegal ones. Documentation may also help the practice fight unemployment claims if the practice records show an employee was disciplined and terminated due to misconduct or for cause.[11]

There are several best practices for documentation. First, establish a companywide policy of avoiding comments or discussions related to job performance in texts or emails as these could be used later during legal proceedings. Be sure to thoroughly investigate any claims of poor job performance or violations of company policy to ensure that any discipline or termination is justified and supported by facts.[12] It's critical to retain documentation of all employee communications about job performance. This includes keeping a record of feedback conversations, accountability meetings, job evaluations, write-ups for poor job performance and all warnings issued for misconduct or inferior job performance.

Written documentation for employee communications needs to be consistent and include the following:

- Date, time, and location
- Statement of which company policy or rule was violated
- Reference any previous write-ups for the same offense
- What discipline is given-e.g., verbal warning, written warning
- Expectations for job improvement and any corrective action employee must take
- Timeline to show progress and consequences if employee fails to meet expectations
- Employee signature with date and witness signature if employee fails to sign[13]

Compliance with Laws

Most employees work according to what is termed "at-will employment" meaning the employee can quit at any time and employers can fire someone at any time without notice as long as it isn't done for an illegal reason. Your employee manual should include an at-will employment disclaimer statement that employees are working at will and that nothing in the handbook constitutes a contract. In addition, if your disciplinary policy refers to a progressive discipline policy, you must clearly state the business has the discretion to skip or alter these steps as deemed appropriate. Otherwise, an employee could claim that you are contractually obligated to follow the disciplinary protocol as outlined in the manual.[14]

At will employees are protected by numerous federal laws from being terminated for illegal reasons. These include laws such as Title VII of the Civil Rights Act of 1964, the Age Discrimination in Employment Act (ADEA), the Fair Labor Standards Act (FLSA) and the Americans with Disabilities Act (ADA). The ADA requires employers to make reasonable accommodations for employees that may include changes to the physical work environment or the way a job is usually performed so team members with a disability can continue to perform their job duties. This can be a tricky area for managers working with employees who develop a disability and may need accommodation. In addition to all federal laws, managers should familiarize themselves with all applicable state laws that protect employees from wrongful termination. Whenever questions arise regarding issues related to employee job performance and the possibility of discrimination, managers should seek legal counsel.

When addressing employee absences, be careful to abide by all federal and state laws that protect employee leave. For companies with 50 or more employees, the Family and Medical Leave Act requires up to 12 weeks of unpaid medical leave. But managers need to be aware that their state laws may require sick leave even if they have less than 50 employees. Some of the more obvious leave policies are for voting leave, military leave, and pregnancy disability leave. But laws also protect employees for absences related to family and medical leave, domestic violence, parental leave and leave to engage in a child's school activities.[15]

CONDUCTING PERFORMANCE REVIEWS

The employee performance review, which is also called an appraisal or evaluation, is a formal assessment by management of the strengths and weaknesses of employees' job performance. Managers conduct performance reviews to provide feedback on how well employees are meeting job expectations and to outline a plan for improvement when needed. Traditionally, companies hold employee review sessions once or twice a year to keep team members informed on how they're doing. Performance evaluations are important, but they're not a replacement for regular feedback and accountability meetings. In fact, in recognition of the value of on-going feedback, some organizations are moving away from the standard annual review process to monthly or quarterly reviews that focus on feedback.

The greatest challenge associated with the annual or bi-annual review process is finding time to complete reviews for the entire team. This can be a significant undertaking for managers with large teams who may find it difficult to complete reviews in a timely manner. The problem with being behind schedule is employees don't get the feedback or raises they deserve. Which leads to another challenge of reviews--that they are frequently tied to raises. Ideally, the review process should be independent of decisions about compensation. Otherwise, employees may go into a review expecting a raise, be disappointed if they don't receive one, and focus more on their compensation than their job performance. The other problem with raises being associated with a review is managers often feel they need to give a raise and may fall into the trap of increasing wages for an underperforming employee.

Another challenge with infrequent reviews occurs if managers don't keep thorough documentation on employees' job performance. It can be difficult to remember details related to someone's job performance from the prior 6-12 months. This leads to more subjective rather than objective assessments. To avoid this problem, managers and supervisors can schedule regular feedback sessions with their direct reports and keep written documentation for these meetings. Then when it's time for formal reviews, there is an accurate record of job performance from the previous year.

Develop a Consistent Process

Regardless of whether your practice evaluates employees using a traditional process of annual reviews or one based on quarterly feedback sessions, you need a consistent protocol to ensure reviews are fair for everyone. One way to schedule reviews on time, is to spread them out over the year based on employees' hire date rather than trying to finish all reviews in one month. You can also stagger meetings if you're doing quarterly reviews. When scheduling reviews, be sure to hold all meetings in private, free from distractions, and that the same amount of time is allocated for all team members.

To implement a consistent process, decide who will review employees and how. In small practices, the manager and practice owner are typically the only ones to evaluate employees. For larger practices, it makes sense to gather evaluations from supervisors and most or all veterinarians who work with an employee. This helps create a more balanced assessment with feedback from multiple practice leaders. It's also beneficial to have employees complete a self-evaluation. This encourages team members to critically think about their job performance before their review. And when managers read self-reviews, they'll know ahead of the meeting if an employee is overly critical of their work or if they have an inflated opinion of how well they're doing.

Some organizations conduct 360-degree reviews whereby everyone on the team reviews every employee. The basis for this process is to create a more complete assessment by having everyone provide feedback on their peers and manager's job performance. But there are drawbacks to 360-degree reviews. One is that team members may feel resentful or hurt by feedback from co-workers especially in small practices where it's hard to maintain confidentiality. Moreover, if employees aren't adequately coached on how to provide objective feedback, they may demonstrate favoritism when reviewing their peers or rank them lower if they perceive they're competing for job roles.

To maintain a consistent review protocol, use written review forms that are the same format for each job position. Ideally, review forms should mirror the employee's job description. It isn't reasonable to address job performance without looking at the job description and asking the question, "is someone successfully performing their duties?" Many standard review forms focus primarily on soft skills and don't include sufficient evaluations for the level of proficiency of hard skills. It's important to assess soft skills such as communication, initiative, and problem-solving capabilities as well as whether a team member adheres to the practice's core values. But practices also need to fully evaluate an employee's technical skills. For example, veterinary technicians and assistants, may be evaluated on how effectively they can set catheters, draw blood, take radiographs, and provide exceptional patient care. CSRs may be evaluated on how well they follow scheduling guidelines, properly enter data into the PMS, process client payments, and their abilities to schedule appointments correctly. By matching review forms to job descriptions, you ensure team members are reviewed based on their job performance of the duties they were hired to do.

Review forms generally have some sort of rating system. A common method is to use a 5-point ranking where 1= Unacceptable, 2=Needs Improvement, 3=Expected, 4=Exceeds Expectations, and 5=Outstanding. Be sure to instruct reviewers to avoid bias and maintain a consistent approach to how they rank employees. Dick Grote, author of the book *How to be Good at Performance Appraisals*, advocates for using a simplified, faster approach where reviewers chose the response of Do More, Do Less or Continue Just as You Are. Then managers can easily focus on items ranked Do More and Do Less.[16] Regardless of which rating system you use, ask reviewers to give specific examples of both positive and negative feedback to best help employees understand the reasons why they received their rankings.

Communication Best Practices

Employees tend to dread reviews because of the uncertainty of not knowing what feedback they will hear. One way managers can promote a positive culture is to set a favorable tone during review meetings, so employees feel as comfortable as possible and know what to expect. Here are some best practices when holding reviews:

- Remind employees the goal for performance reviews is to let them know what they need to keep doing, what they can do to enhance their job performance, and any corrective actions they must take to improve. Transparency is important, so explain the process that was used for their performance evaluation.
- Be professional and direct. Exhibit professionalism by approaching the review as an opportunity to help employees; put aside personal emotions. Include information about poor job performance or lack of accountability.

- Be empathetic. Even negative feedback can be delivered with empathy.
- Tie job performance behaviors to the core values of the business.
- Take care not to sugar coat or bury the message when employees aren't meeting job expectations.
- During the review or at the end, solicit feedback from employees and inquire whether they have any questions.
- Include a clear action plan. When employees exceed expectations, the plan may simply be to continue the excellent work and to pursue further growth opportunities. When action is needed to improve job performance, employees need to know specifically what they need to do. Telling someone they need to be a better team player, or they need to focus on improving their communication skills is just setting them up for failure if they don't have a plan to accomplish these goals. (Employee development plans are covered in Chapter 6 on Employee Retention.)

DISCIPLINE AND PERFORMANCE IMPROVEMENT PLANS

Using discipline to improve job performance isn't a good plan if it's the primary method used to increase employee accountability and develop a positive culture. No one wants to work at a business where there is fear of "being written up" or where co-workers advocate for making sure people "get written up" whenever they make mistakes. In this type of culture, trust is low and the approach to discipline seems punitive. Rather than immediately jumping to discipline, it's much better to provide regular feedback and manage by core values to enhance employee job performance.

Of course, discipline is warranted when there is a flagrant disregard for policies or violation of the code of conduct. Discipline is also appropriate when employees demonstrate consistent inferior job performance even after being given negative feedback and guidance on what they need to do to improve. Every practice needs a disciplinary policy, so employees understand the justifications for discipline and the consequences of poor performance. The goal of a disciplinary policy is to eliminate bad behavior and to give people an opportunity to improve thereby retaining good employees. This leads to the preservation of a high-performing culture of accountability and teamwork.

Progressive Discipline

Progressive discipline is a process of discipline where employees who demonstrate poor conduct or job performance receive a series of reprimands starting with a verbal warning followed by a written warning and then a final warning or suspension followed by termination if corrective action isn't taken. The purpose of progressive discipline is to treat every employee fairly and give them one or more chances to improve their job performance. In addition, the documentation associated with progressive discipline is used to show employers afforded employees the opportunity to eliminate problem behaviors, abide by policies and meet job expectations.

Sometimes managers don't fully understand how to effectively use progressive discipline with employees. The system doesn't have to be rigid; there are no rules that you must give one verbal warning, one written warning and then terminate an employee. You may elect to give multiple verbal warnings and multiple written warnings. But if the warnings never lead to termination, then the system doesn't work because ultimately there is no consequence for unacceptable job performance. Tardiness is an excellent example of how this happens. Managers who need team members, especially talented ones, are usually hesitant to fire someone for tardiness even if they have been given multiple warnings.

Another misconception is thinking you must go through the progressive discipline protocol for all problem behaviors. If an employee has a major offense that violates the hospital's core values or the code of conduct, managers may decide immediate termination is the best course of action. Regardless of whether a verbal or written warning is issued, it is paramount that managers document these communications with employees as noted in the previous section on documentation.

How To Write an Effective Performance Improvement Plan

With infractions such as tardiness or a single violation of a company policy such as not abiding by the dress code, managers can easily communicate with negative feedback or a warning about what action needs to be taken. Show up for work on time and dress in accordance with the dress code policy. But what about those circumstances when employees aren't meeting job expectations and may have job performance problems in multiple areas? The underlying cause of the difficulty could be personal problems, lack of training, poor job fit, suboptimal motivation, or a combination of factors. Regardless of the known or suspected reasons for poor performance, in these instances, managers need to create a written performance improvement plan (PIP) that outlines specific examples of poor job performance and what actions the employee must take to keep their job. (See Figure 5.2: Performance Improvement Plan.)

For a PIP to be effective, managers need to have a genuine desire and willingness to help an employee improve their job performance. A PIP is appropriate when managers aren't sure if a team member can excel but want to give them every opportunity to succeed. But the process isn't meant to be used as a means to terminate an employee.[17] When there is a desire to ultimately terminate someone, the disciplinary process should be used to document poor job performance, not a PIP.

The PIP should be a comprehensive, written document that includes examples of poor job performance, clear job expectations, any training the employee must complete, and specific details about what improvements must be made. For example, an underperforming veterinary assistant might have a PIP that includes these four goals: 1) eliminate tardiness, 2) demonstrate proficiency with client education about preventive care, 3) properly prepare patients for surgery without supervision, 4) accurately perform in-house laboratory tests. Each goal needs to list available resources for training and deadlines for completion. In addition, the PIP should include a timeline for meetings with a manager or supervisor and the consequences of failing to meet all the objectives. These details are important so employees understand they must improve their job performance in all areas within a defined amount of time.

Figure 5.2: Performance Improvement Plan

Performance Improvement Plan (PIP) - Confidential

Employee Name:

Title:

Date:

The purpose of this Performance Improvement Plan (PIP) is to define areas of concern regarding your job performance. It also affords you the opportunity to demonstrate improvement and your commitment to keeping your current job position. This document specifies any gaps in your work performance, lack of accountability, and failure to demonstrate progress toward goals. It also re-establishes job expectations and outlines the necessary action steps to improve your job performance.

Areas of Concern:

Summary of Previous Job Performance Meetings:

Goals/Actions to Improve:

Figure 5.2: Performance Improvement Plan (continued)

Target Date to meet each goal/show improvement:

Target date for performance improvement:

Next steps/meeting dates to review progress:

Acknowledgement

Employee Signature: _____ Date: _____

Supervisor Signature: _____ Date: _____

Note: This performance improvement plan is not intended to be an employment contract or guarantee of continuing employment.

Progress review notes:

Comments:

Employee Feedback/Comments:

Review accepted by:

Employee Signature: _____ Date: _____

Review completed by:

Supervisor Signature: _____ Date: _____

TERMINATION

While no one likes to terminate an employee, practice owners and managers are sometimes remiss in not acting soon enough to let go of underperforming team members. Worse yet, some businesses hang on to toxic employees far too long before they fire them. Here are common reasons why practices don't take action to terminate employees with unacceptable job performance:

- An employee has valuable skills
- It's difficult to find a replacement
- They've worked at the practice for a long time
- Fear that clients who love the employee may be upset and leave the practice

- The employee is well liked by the rest of the team and/or management
- The employee is in a protected class
- There is a lack of documentation regarding poor job performance
- Conflict avoidance and fear of confrontation; not wanting to feel bad for firing someone
- Employees show temporary improvement and then backslide which leads to a roller coaster of lows and highs regarding job performance

Interestingly, veterinary practice teams rarely report that the feared outcomes of termination are a problem. In fact, it's not uncommon for everyone on the team to feel relieved when someone with bad behavior or who isn't pulling their weight is terminated. Having said this, managers need to use caution when making decisions about termination and follow a consistent, fair process. When grounds for termination exists such as a grievous violation of the code of conduct, it isn't necessary to implement progressive disciplinary procedures. But in other situations, employees should be given every opportunity to improve their job performance as outlined in progressive discipline warnings or a PIP. As stated previously, it is always prudent to consult an attorney if there are concerns about a discrimination or wrongful termination claim.

Once the decision has been made to terminate an employee, it should be done respectfully. Termination meetings must occur in private and there should always be a witness. While this can be awkward for both parties, it avoids a "he said, she said" situation if there is a legal claim later and the presence of a second person may discourage angry outbursts. Ideally, it is best to hold termination meetings early in the workweek toward the end of the day, so people have time to take action that week to secure new employment. This can also help with privacy and make it easier for employees to gracefully leave the hospital. Termination meetings should be short. Give the employee a brief description of why they are being fired and avoid any arguments. Inform the employee when they will receive their final paycheck and request that they return any hospital property.

SUMMARY

All practices need multiple human resource management procedures aimed at enhancing and evaluating job performance. One of the most beneficial methods to help employees excel and contribute to the business is to manage by core values. By referencing the hospital's core values when giving negative and positive feedback, practice owners and managers can develop their desired culture. Other essential components of human resource management communications include clearly establishing job expectations and responsibilities when delegating work and following up with consistent feedback. Managers also need to address lack of accountability when it occurs. This starts by identifying underlying causes for the problem and putting plans in place to help employees meet (and hopefully exceed) job expectations.

In addition to having an employee policy manual, managers need to conduct fair and consistent employee evaluations, so team members know what they're doing well and how they need to improve. Communications about job performance including employee reviews, accountability meetings, PIPs, disciplinary warnings, and termination meetings should all be documented. This helps avoid discrimination claims and lawsuits.

CHAPTER 6

Employee Retention

Employee retention refers to whether employees stay with a company rather than seeking a job elsewhere. It also refers to the strategies companies use to retain team members. The opposite of retention is turnover. It's generally accepted that it's better to retain employees than to have to find new ones. In part this is because of the cost associated with recruitment which includes the manager's time spent on hiring, advertising expenses, training costs, and the loss of productivity that may result when an employee leaves the practice. Moreover, there is the additional cost that is harder to quantify associated with the loss of knowledge and skill sets of a talented employee.

You can calculate the employee retention rate by looking at the total number of employees at the beginning of a time period minus the employees who left and then dividing this number by the total number of employees. Here is an example:

25 total employees-2 employees lost = 23 employees retained

23 employees/25 employees = .92 X 100 = 92% retention[1]

Employee retention rates vary by industry, but most companies consider an employee retention rate of 90% to be desirable. The retention rate decreases if employee turnover is high. People may leave jobs for reasons such as retirement, changing careers, and relocation. But often employee turnover is related to job satisfaction and compensation. If someone can easily get a higher paying job, one that affords them greater opportunities, and offers a better work environment, then they're more likely to leave. In veterinary medicine, employee turnover has also been linked to the stress associated with job roles which can lead to compassion fatigue and burnout. As noted in Chapter 3, it can be difficult to find qualified team members for a veterinary hospital. Therefore, it's advisable for managers to do everything they can to minimize turnover of talented employees.

Bear in mind some level of turnover is good. The goal isn't just to keep employees but rather to retain excellent team members. It doesn't do the business any good to retain employees who lack accountability, create conflict, or are poor performers. It's beneficial for businesses to occasionally add new employees with a fresh perspective. Some amount of turnover helps to avoid stagnant cultures characterized by entrenched thinking, reluctance to change, lack of creativity, and a lack of diversity. New employees often bring in new knowledge, ideas, and skill sets.

Table 6.1: Retention Strategies

Retention Strategies	Description
Compensation and benefits	• Competitive compensation and benefits • Equitable wages • Opportunities to increase pay (e.g., raises, bonuses, profit-sharing)
Meaningful work	• Doing work that has clear purpose and value • Community involvement
Manager relationship	• Managers give feedback • Managers care about the team and ensure employees feel valued • Managers show appreciation
Trusted leadership	• Leaders are ethical • Leadership communications are honest and transparent
Employee development	• Opportunity for advancement • Opportunity to learn and grow • Ability to use skills and knowledge
Culture of well-being	• Leaders promote both physical and emotional well-being • Policies and activities exist that promote well-being
Diversity and inclusion	• Recruitment strategies promote diversity • DE&I policy exists and is followed • Leadership actively promotes inclusion • All policies and opportunities support equity
Employee empowerment	• Team members have some level of autonomy • Employees allowed to make decisions • Leaders coach team members to higher levels of job performance
Work environment	• Positive, happy place to work • Cohesive teams • Team building activities

It's a good idea to periodically evaluate the business's retention and turnover rates. If a significant number of employees are leaving this may indicate something isn't going well; either people aren't paid appropriately, or they aren't happy. When recruiting and hiring team members, practices need to offer competitive compensation packages. Employers also need to continue to pay competitive wages to retain team members. But aside from compensation, the best way to retain employees is create a positive culture where people enjoy coming to work. In this chapter, we further explore how to create a desirable work environment and increase employee retention by focusing on increasing employee engagement and team building. (See Figure 6.1 for an overview of retention strategies.)

UNDERSTANDING EMPLOYEE ENGAGEMENT

The Gallup organization defines engaged employees as those who are both enthusiastic and committed to their work.[2] Put another way, engaged employees are those who are satisfied or happy with their jobs and are contributing to the company. Conversely, disengaged employees have some level of unhappiness or suboptimal motivation about their job or the work environment. Note that an employee may be talented and highly productive (thus contributing to the company) but be disengaged because they're unhappy in their job. In this instance, disengagement might show up as negativity, lack of teamwork, or conflict with co-workers. On the other hand, an employee may be generally satisfied with their job (maybe due to high compensation or a preferred work schedule) but be disengaged and thus contribute minimally to the success of the business. In this instance, disengagement might show up as lack of initiative, resistance to change, or a drop in job performance. High levels of employee disengagement can negatively affect morale, accountability, and team productivity.

Engagement Surveys

One of the ways organizations can assess the level of engagement is to survey employees. Companies with an HR department have historically used an annual employee survey to gain insight about how employees feel about their jobs. To be an effective measure of engagement, surveys need to be designed to determine the level of dedication, passion and motivation employees have for their jobs and the business they work for.[3] The Gallup organization has studied employee engagement for many years and regularly publishes data on the level of engagement for U.S. workers. The questions developed by Gallup assess the level of engagement based on twelve elements of employee engagement they've identified as predictors of high team performance.[4] The questions focus on whether an employee's needs are met, whether they feel connected to the team, and whether they have an opportunity to do what they do best and grow professionally.

There are pros and cons of doing engagement surveys. They can be helpful if businesses act on employees' feedback. Let's say, for example, a survey reveals the majority of team members don't feel they receive recognition for their work or don't understand their job expectations. If the leadership team addresses these concerns by clarifying job expectations and giving more positive feedback, employees will likely feel heard. But if engagement is low and no action is taken, employees may be left feeling as if the survey was a waste of time and that management doesn't really care about what they think.

An alternative to annual engagement surveys is to use more frequent pulse surveys to check in with employees and assess how they feel about their work. Because pulse surveys usually have 10 or fewer questions and employees complete the survey online, it's a fast way to solicit team feedback.[5] Managers who want to use engagement surveys are wise to research which questions have been shown to be most enlightening and may want to consider using an outside company or consultant to administer the survey.

Exit Surveys and Stay Interviews

Employers can use exit surveys to gain feedback from departing employees so the business can better understand their level of job satisfaction and any factors that may have contributed to the employee's decision to leave. Ideally, team members who resign will convey valuable information practice leaders can use to understand what's working well at the practice and make improvements if needed. There are several challenges with exit surveys. First, employees who are leaving may not want to take time to complete a survey so the simpler they are, the better. Another issue is that employees who want to maintain relations with the business and/or receive a positive job reference may be reluctant to disclose anything negative on an exit survey. And lastly, if an employee clearly resigns because they weren't happy, it can be awkward or uncomfortable to ask them to fill out a survey.

Given the limitations of exit surveys, businesses are increasingly using stay surveys as a proactive way to increase employee retention of talented employees. The best way to do a stay survey is to hold an informal one-on-one meeting with an employee to explore their views on their job and the work environment. Approach the meeting similarly to an interview meaning the goal is to primarily ask questions to solicit feedback from employees. The key to success for a stay interview is to act on the information the employee presents.[6] For example, if someone indicates they don't feel they can advance in the company, the manager will need to work with the team member to identify opportunities for them to learn and grow.

When conducting stay interviews, strive to put employees at ease and use a standard set of questions designed to understand why employees may or may not choose to stay. Examples of good stay interview questions include:

- What is the best part (or worst part) of working here?
- What would you like to do that you're not currently doing?
- What would you like to learn more about?
- What can I do more of or less of as your manager?
- What might tempt you to leave?[7]

Managers that want to do employee surveys and stay interviews should implement protocols outlining how and when the management tools will be utilized. This helps to ensure these activities are consistent and equitable for the entire team. Regardless of whether you use engagement surveys, exit surveys, or stay interviews, remember that the goal is to look for early signs that employees aren't happy so you can take action to enhance employee retention.

Extrinsic vs. Intrinsic Rewards

To better understand employee engagement, it's important to recognize how extrinsic and intrinsic rewards affect levels of engagement. Extrinsic rewards are tangible rewards given to employees such as a pay raise, bonus, plaque, or favorable benefits. Compensation is a critical factor for employee recruitment and team members need to be paid fairly. But once employees are hired, extrinsic rewards don't typically lead to higher levels of employee engagement. While extrinsic rewards are desirable, they tend to have a short-term effect on employee motivation and engagement.[8]

On the other hand, intrinsic rewards are directly correlated with employee retention because they are high drivers of engagement. We think of intrinsic rewards as the feelings we have when we do a good job. This might be pride in a job well done, a sense of accomplishment when learning new skills or a sense of fulfillment for being able to help someone. Research shows employees are more motivated and engaged at work when the following four intrinsic rewards are present: a sense of meaningfulness, choice, competence, and progress. What this means is employees are more likely to be engaged if they feel they're doing work that has purpose, they have some ownership over how they do their work, they have the skills needed to do a good job, and that their work efforts make a difference or allow for growth.[9]

EMPLOYEE ENGAGEMENT STRATEGIES

Implementing specific employee engagement strategies is the best way to increase employee retention. When considering what strategies to focus on, remember the goal isn't just to retain employees but rather to retain high performers who are eager to come to work and will contribute to the practice's success. Research from Gallup across multiple industries in many countries shows the clear relationship between employee engagement and business outcomes. The research shows a decrease in turnover and an increase in customer engagement, productivity, and profitability with higher levels of engagement. It's also noteworthy that employee well-being is much higher with organizations that have higher employee engagement.[10] (See Figure 6.1: Benefits of High Employee Engagement.)

Figure 6.1: Benefits of High Employee Engagement

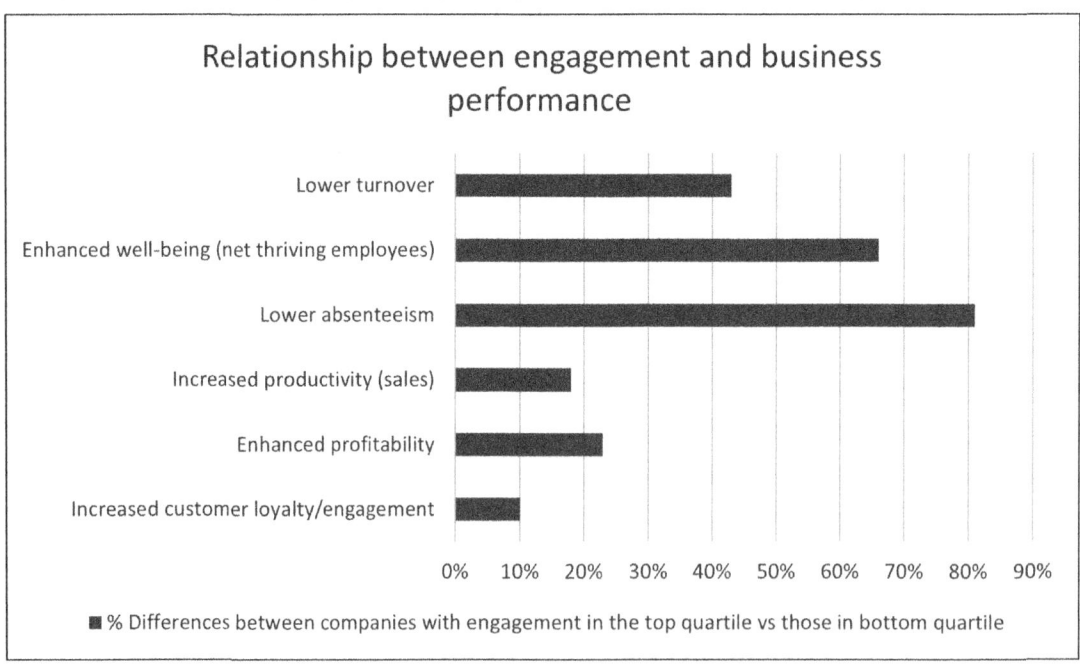

Source: Adapted from Gallup's report on The Powerful Relationship Between Employee Engagement and Team Performance, https://www.gallup.com/workplace/321032/employee-engagement-meta-analysis-brief.aspx, October 2020.

Clearly enhancing employee engagement is good for team members and for the business. Let's take a look at specific strategies that increase employees' intrinsic rewards (and thus engagement).

Enhancing Employee-Manager Relationships

The relationship employees have with their boss can make or break whether they're engaged at work and whether they want to continue to work for a company. Depending on the practice size and management structure, veterinary employees may report to a supervisor, office manager, practice manager, hospital administrator, regional director, or directly to the practice owner. All these members of the leadership team need to know how to foster positive relationships with their direct reports. Moreover, they need to understand how their actions can help increase employees' intrinsic rewards and job satisfaction.

According to a research report by the Society of Human Resource Management, employees identified respectful treatment of all employees at all levels as one of the top five contributors to job satisfaction.[11] Team members have a strong desire to work for someone they like and respect. It's easy to identify what employees don't like about supervisors and the characteristics of a toxic boss. No one likes a manager that yells, criticizes, blames, ignores, harasses, micromanages, gossips, or plays favorites. When subjected to these types of behaviors, employees increasingly find it difficult to stay in their job position. But sometimes a manager has a negative behavior and may not even realize how their actions affect team members. Which brings us to the question: What makes for a positive relationship? What should managers focus on?

The hallmark of a good employee-manager relationship is excellent communication so reflect on how well you connect with team members. In earlier chapters you learned about honing communication skills such as active listening, asking good questions, and giving effective feedback. You also learned about how to foster a positive culture with communications that focus on core values and promoting inclusion. All these communications help increase employee engagement and retention. In Chapter 7 on Communication Challenges and Solutions, you'll learn more about how to build positive relationships with team members by becoming adept at handling difficult team communications and promoting self-leadership.

With respect to increasing employee engagement, perhaps the most important aspect of communication is making sure employees know you genuinely care about them. Expressing sincere appreciation to team members on a regular basis is one of the best ways to show you care. Note the difference between appreciation and feedback. Feedback focuses on an employee's behavior as it relates to aspects of their job performance. Appreciation focuses on the person and their value. When giving positive feedback, the primary purpose is to describe specific observed behaviors you want to recognize or reward. When giving appreciation, you validate a person's worth and show you're paying attention. You might say "I appreciate your kindness and thoughtfulness."[12]

Building Trust with The Team

When people think of trust, they think about the actions and behaviors that make someone trustworthy. Trustworthy people do what they say they will and act with good intentions. Employees want to work for leaders they can trust. Without trust, team members become uneasy because they don't have confidence in their manager or other practice leaders to do the right thing and act in the best interest of the team. This lack of trust can lead to low levels of engagement for some employees or the entire team. (See Figure 1.4: Leadership actions that build or break down trust in Chapter 1 for more about actions that build trust.)

David Horsager, author of *Trusted Leader: 8 Pillars That Drive Results*, has studied the link between trust and employee retention. His research shows that trusted leadership helps attract and retain the best talent. He cites that 64% of people indicated transparent communication and keeping promises were the most important actions employers take that increase how long they stay with their company. Interestingly, his work reveals that 76% of people believe ongoing development and training would help them trust their employer more.[13]

One way managers sometimes unknowingly break down trust is associated with employee compensation. The need to offer competitive compensation as a strategy to attract and hire excellent job candidates was presented in Chapter 3 on Recruiting and Hiring Team Members. One of the pitfalls related to compensation and retention can occur when a new employee is hired at a higher wage than other employees in the company who are doing the same job. Team members who find out someone with less tenure or experience is making more than them usually feel angry and unappreciated. Even if managers agree to a raise when confronted by an unhappy employee, trust breaks down and hurt feelings may persist.

To avoid this scenario and keep good employees, develop a transparent and consistent compensation strategy. The best way to ensure fairness with compensation is to establish criteria for pay ranges for each job position. Evaluate pay scales annually to be sure team members are paid competitive wages for the industry and the area where the practice is located. Additionally, paying employees based on performance helps to retain excellent employees. Practices can develop criteria for team members to increase their pay based on their level of skill sets and knowledge. Managers with a compensation strategy can give cost of living raises and merit increases as appropriate based on the practice's compensation guidelines.

There are multiple communications that help to build trust with the team, some of which have been presented in earlier chapters. An essential communication your learned in Chapter 2 is to provide clarity regarding the organization's vision, mission, core values, and goals as well as job expectations. Employees inherently have more trust when they know what an organization stands for and how they fit in. Practice leaders that manage by core values and use the core values as a roadmap for behaviors and actions further build trust with their team. Another critical communication to build a high trust culture is to keep employees informed. Therefore, it's imperative to be honest and straightforward with communications. This is particularly true in times of crisis. Business owners and managers that communicated openly with their teams and explained the reason for all changes during the COVID-19 pandemic built higher levels of trust.

Recognize too, that managers build trust simply by competently performing their job duties. This is because employees easily lose confidence in managers who exhibit indecisiveness or seem uncomfortable doing their job. This doesn't mean managers need to know everything, but they do need to project self-confidence and let employees know when they will have answers or take action. If a piece of equipment is broken, for example, team members reasonably want it to be fixed and know when it will be repaired. Another part of being a competent manager is to be consistent. This means being a consistently positive leader and a reliable manager. It means consistently striving to affect positive change and following through on all promises. And it means avoiding favoritism, ensuring that everyone adheres to the hospital policies, and treating everyone fairly.

Consider Generational Differences

Most veterinary practices employ team members from three to four different generations. However, it's noteworthy that as of 2021 the two youngest generations, Generation Z and millennials, account for 46% of the U.S full-time workers.[14] The Pew Research Center considers anyone born 1981-1996 to be a millennial and anyone born from 1997 forward to be in the Gen Z group.[15] Given the increasing large number of younger people in the workforce, it's wise for employers to understand what younger employees want. According to the Gallup organization, what Gen Z and millennials most want is a business that cares about their physical and emotional well-being. These two generations also place significant importance on working for an organization that promotes diversity and inclusion as well as one where leaders are open and transparent.[16]

In 2016, Monster, one of the leading job-placement companies, reported results from their Multi-Generational Survey focusing on what Generation Z is looking for from employers. (See Figure 6.2: What Gen Z Wants in the Workplace.) The results reinforce how important it is to discuss the core values of the business and how every employee contributes to the meaningful work of helping pets and people. The survey also shows the need to help younger team members grow and advance to higher wages.

Figure 6.2: What Gen Z Wants in the Workplace

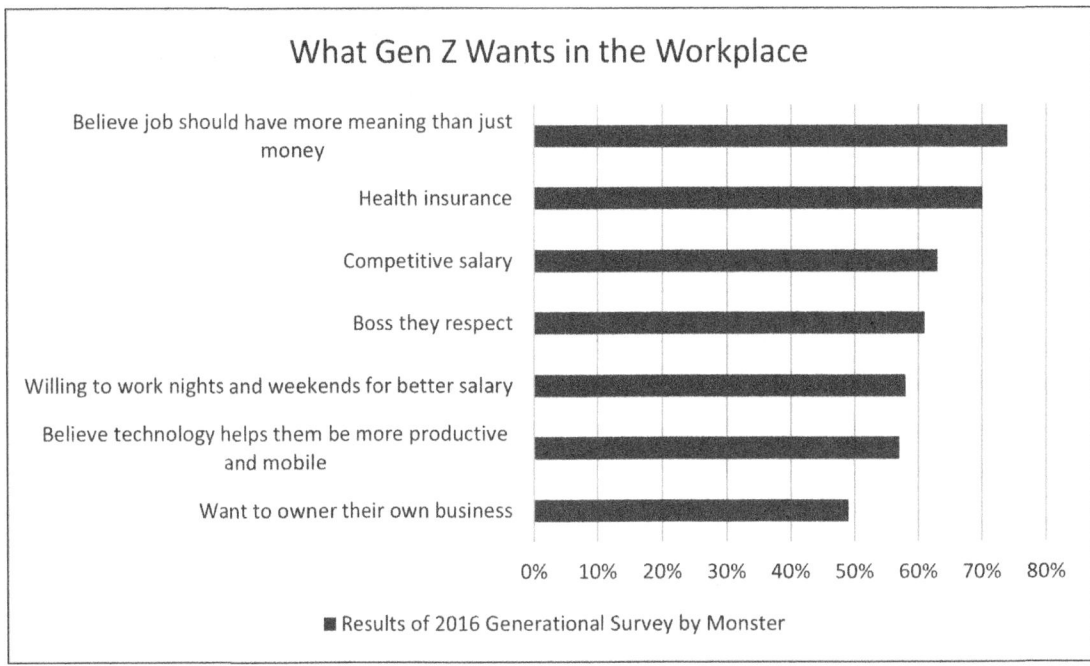

Source: Adapted from Monster's Multi-Generational Survey. https://www.monstersoftwaresolutions.com/docs/genz/monster_genz_report.pdf.

To retain younger generations, begin by looking at the business's policies, operations, and culture. Then consider the following questions. Does the practice have core values and defined behaviors that align with the values? Does the business have a DE&I policy that is followed? Is there a defined code of professional conduct? Does the practice use the latest technology for client and internal communications? Does the practice have a strong presence on social media? Do managers seek to gain feedback from team members and make sure everyone has a voice during team meetings? Is there a process to coach younger team members and make sure they have development opportunities? And very importantly, what programs are available that promote and support well-being?

Employee Development

Employee development is the process of helping team members gain knowledge, skills, and abilities. Employee development programs promote learning and growth for all team members regardless of their current level of expertise. Developing the talent of employees is a proven driver of employee engagement and retention. This is because employees feel valued, and their intrinsic rewards increase when they can successfully do their job. When people have opportunities to use their skills and excel at work, they are more likely to stay with the company.

Employee development programs should be differentiated from the employee review process. Often employee reviews end with a discussion about goals that focuses on what employees aren't doing well. There's nothing inherently wrong with talking about goals during the review process but these conversations tend to focus on employees' shortcomings and frequently don't include a detailed plan for how to achieve the desired goal. Moreover, sometimes the goals discussed relate to a lack of accountability instead of development and may be more appropriate for a PIP. Employee reviews look back at prior job performance whereas employee development is a forward-thinking process that focuses on future possibilities of what team members can learn and how they can grow.

Younger generations, in particular, have a strong desire for development and may leave practices if they aren't challenged or feel there is no chance for advancement. Surveys by Gallup reveal 59% of millennial job seekers want opportunities to learn and grow. And 50% of millennials report that chances for advancement are extremely important to them.[17] Generation Z, the newest generation to enter the workforce, also has an interest in employee development. This generation is looking for stability and opportunities for advancement in the workplace. Studies show that 61% of Gen Z indicated they would stay at a company for more than 10 years but that they want to be able to get ahead based on their job performance, not how long they have held their job.[18]

But what about those employees who seem to have no interest in gaining more knowledge or learning new skills? If you face this situation, strive to determine factors that may be related to a team member's disinterest. Sometimes disengaged team members don't seem interested in learning even though development may be the very strategy that can increase their level of engagement. So, it's critical to encourage all employees to pursue education and professional growth. One of the keys to effective employee development programs is to work with the willing but don't overlook the talent and potential of all team members. Reasons for lack of employee motivation and why people resist change are presented in the next chapter.

Employee development is a two-way process that involves both employees and the organization. Development plans need to focus on ensuring employees gain the requisite skills they need to be successful in their position. This is especially true for new hires and inexperienced team members. But you also want to meet with team members to discuss their specific interests and desires for learning. One veterinary assistant, for example, might be interested in nutrition and patient care while another might be more interested in behavior and developing their laboratory skills. One CSR might be primarily motivated to hone their client communication skills while another is interested in learning more about how to assist with the hospital's social media program. When you understand what type of professional development team members desire, you have a much greater likelihood of increasing employee engagement.

Challenges might surface if an employee wants to focus their development on job duties they don't seem to have the talent for. For example, a team member might not have the talent to excel in surgery which requires careful attention to detail, the ability to monitor anesthesia and specific patient care skills. Alternatively, an employee might shy away from developing skills related to job responsibilities they don't enjoy but where everyone needs to excel such as enhancing client communication skills. In these instances, it's the job of managers to help team members see where their strengths are and that not everyone has the same aptitude. At the same time, you need to help employees understand they can't always pick and choose their job duties based on personal preferences. Remember too, that employee development goals need to align with hospital goals. This means the knowledge and expertise gained by achieving goals should benefit the business, not just the employee.

Training is the cornerstone of employee development programs. Chapter 4 on Team Training outlines how to implement effective training programs. But having training programs doesn't necessarily mean the business has an effective employee development program. To be a successful engagement strategy, employee development needs to be an on-going, organized, comprehensive program that helps team members reach specific goals.

Ideally, every team member should have a written development plan that they review with their supervisor in a face-to-face meeting at least quarterly if not monthly. For larger practices, it makes sense for department supervisors to facilitate development meetings rather than the practice manager. All employee development meetings need to be documented so managers can track employees' progress toward their goals. Ongoing discussions about development should center on what employees have learned, what new skills they've developed, increases in ability, and what challenges they may have encountered. Let's say a CSR has a goal of enhancing their phone skills. It would be important to define their current skill set and what new communication skills they will practice. A review of specific recorded calls could be used to assess proficiency, identify successes, and discuss what the employee needs to do differently to improve. Remember, development plans need to specify a timetable and deadlines for achievement of goals. (See Figure 6.3 for an employee development form.)

Technician Utilization

One of the most essential retention strategies for credentialed veterinary technicians is to ensure they're empowered to use all their skills and knowledge. Therefore, it makes sense to routinely assess whether the practice is effectively utilizing its credentialled technicians. Multiple organizations have identified that the underutilization of technicians is a concern for the profession. In 2019, the AVMA formed the AVMA Task Force on Veterinary Technician Utilization to evaluate this issue. In 2020, their report was received by the AVMA Board of Directors. The group's recommendations included initiatives to use surveys and data to evaluate issues related to availability and attrition of technicians, develop programs to promote the value of technicians, support ongoing research for mental health issues and focus on ways to enhance well-being in the workplace.[19]

Consider these questions to assess whether the practice is effectively using its credentialed technicians:

- Are technicians routinely doing job duties such as cleaning kennels, animal restraint and working as a client service representative?
- Are technicians fully leveraged to assist veterinarians with client education?
- Are technicians afforded opportunities for more advanced continuing education?
- Are the veterinarians in the practice performing services that a credentialed technician could be doing?
- Are technicians regularly performing more advanced skills such as placing urinary catheters, patient monitoring, administration of anesthesia, and bandage applications?
- Are technicians routinely seeing appointments to perform services allowed by the state's practice act?

Figure 6: Employee Development Plan

Employee Developmental Plan

Employee name: _____ Position: _____
Manager/Supervisor: _____ Start Date: _____
Mentor: _____ End Date: _____

Required Core Competencies:
Career goal (short or long-term):
Areas of interest:
Strengths:
Areas for improvement:
Training needs:

Goals Planner

Goal: _____

Action steps	Target date	Completion date
1. _____	_____	_____
2. _____	_____	_____
3. _____	_____	_____

Goal: _____

Action steps	Target date	Completion date
1. _____	_____	_____
2. _____	_____	_____
3. _____	_____	_____

Goal: _____

Action steps	Target date	Completion date
1. _____	_____	_____
2. _____	_____	_____
3. _____	_____	_____

Measurement of Proficiency: Completion date
(e.g., skills test, written quiz, verbal quiz, completion of training,
CE attendance, task completed, new behavior observed)
_____   _____
_____   _____

Resources for assistance:
_____   _____

You can also look at a Veterinary Technician Utilization Assessment tool created by a group of veterinary technician leaders in the profession. It can be used to help determine if credentialled technicians could be used more effectively in the practice (https://vtutilization.com/).

Be sure to actively work with credentialed technicians to create development plans that focus on how they can best use their skills and continue to advance their career. Not only does proper technician utilization enhance retention, it also improves patient care, increases doctor productivity, enhances efficiency, and helps to grow revenues for the business.

Employee Empowerment

Employee empowerment is defined as giving employees the autonomy and responsibility to make decisions. Employees typically have different levels of empowerment based on their job position, skills, level of experience, and how much control managers are willing to give up. The amount of empowerment given to an employee is also based on the amount of trust the organization has in their ability to make good decisions. Associate veterinarians, for example, are fully empowered to treat patients without supervision unless perhaps they're a new graduate. By contrast, a veterinary technician in charge of inventory may be empowered to make decisions on how much to order each week but may be required to seek approval before taking advantage of vendor promotions or adding a new drug to the hospital supply.

Empowerment is an effective employee engagement strategy because it increases the intrinsic reward of choice. Most people have greater job satisfaction if they have some level of control over their work and can make decisions without constantly seeking approval. Empowered employees are more likely to stay in their job because they enjoy the rewards of being a valued team member who can contribute to the success of the business.

To decide how to best empower team members, it's helpful to first recognize the actual level of empowerment current employees may or may not have. Some practice owners and managers think they've empowered their team when in reality that isn't true. To determine how empowered your team is, you can look at the nature of daily interruptions from team members and the questions they routinely ask you. To do this, confidentially conduct the following exercise over one or more weeks.

1. Track all your employee interruptions that necessitate follow-up action or decisions. Here are examples of what employees might say or ask:

- "The centrifuge isn't working properly."
- "Can I post this photo to Facebook?"
- "I don't have anyone to cover Alicia's shift next week."
- "Mrs. Jones isn't happy about her bill. What should I do?"
- "We ran out of 500 mg Cephalexin and Dr. Taylor needs it for a patient going home today."
- "Mr. Smith wants to bring in Jake, but I don't have any open appointments today."

2. Make note of your response. Common responses include:
   - "Ok, I'll take care of it."
   - "I'll help you with this later."
   - "I'll be there in a few minutes."
   - "Please go ask Dr. Taylor what she wants you to do."

3. Note who comes to you with questions or concerns and categorize the interruptions.
   - Is it all team members or just a few?
   - Is there any pattern for the interruptions based on the day or time of day?
   - Are the interruptions relevant or urgent (you must be the person to handle the situation).

4. Evaluate the interruptions. Ask yourself:
   - Why do employees come to me about this situation?
   - Could they have solved this problem or decided on their own what action to take?
   - Why don't they?

The goal of completing the above activity is to figure out if there are opportunities to empower your team more fully. Not only does this increase engagement and retention, it cuts down your interruptions and increases productivity. When assessing the information you gleaned from the exercise, consider the following possible reasons why employees don't act or feel like they aren't empowered to decide what to do:

- Lack of clarity about job responsibilities and job roles
- Hospital protocols aren't clear
- Poor job fit
- Lack of training
- Suboptimal motivation (disengaged)
- Lack of empowerment

Always first consider if lack of training or lack of clarity about job responsibilities are an underlying factor especially with new hires. If multiple team members have the same question or concern, then lack of clarity about protocols or ineffective systems may be to blame. If employees have received sufficient training, then poor job fit, or a lack of engagement may be a problem. And lastly, if team members are capable but don't act, then they simply may not be empowered (or don't think they are).

In looking at the above scenarios, it's clear that an empowered employee should know what to do and could have handled the problems or at least propose a solution. This exercise helps you determine what an employee might need so they can do their job better. In Chapter 5 on Enhancing and Evaluating Job Performance, you learned about effective delegation and how to give feedback. These actions are the foundation for employee empowerment. Therefore, it's always a good idea to evaluate whether the underlying problem with lack of empowerment is related to delegation or feedback. It's easy to fall into the trap of taking care of every issue brought to you by employees but this habit limits empowerment and stifles engagement. Make sure you're giving team members opportunities to contribute. In Chapter 7 you will learn more about how to empower team members by promoting self-leadership and coaching employees to be problem-solvers.

When thinking of employee empowerment, you may feel like you can't empower everyone on the team. After all, some employees don't seem to want autonomy and it may seem like others aren't capable of making decisions on their own. While it's true not everyone wants to be empowered, it's prudent to carefully consider factors that might influence an employee's desire for autonomy such as lack of training or fear of failure. Additionally, a team member might feel management doesn't trust them or will be overly critical of their decisions, so why bother. One way to encourage empowerment is to ask team members what they'd like to be able to do that they currently aren't allowed to do as well as their greatest frustrations at work. This gives you a good idea where to start efforts to increase employee autonomy. It takes time to empower team members, but the benefits of improved efficiency, increased engagement and greater employee retention are well worth the effort.

TEAM BUILDING

Team building is defined as the process of encouraging employees to work well together and usually involves activities designed to promote cooperation.[20] The purpose of team building in the workplace is to promote teamwork, improve internal communication, and help people get to know their co-workers better. Team building activities can also help employees better understand each other, reduce conflict, and promote more creative problem-solving.

Team building isn't the same as scheduling events to show appreciation and have fun. Social activities such as trivia games, staff parties, and a night of bowling are valuable ways to show caring and may improve morale at least temporarily. Team building activities, on the other hand, are more about creating an environment where employees can learn how to better collaborate and reach goals together.

To decide on the best team building activities, consider the primary purpose. Is it just to have fun? Is it to improve listening skills? Or perhaps it is to help a diverse group of team members understand each other better. Here are examples of fun team building activities that promote camaraderie and encourage teamwork:

- Escape room event
- Scavenger hunt
- Interactive games or solving puzzles
- Community service projects
- Organizing an outdoor group activity such as a walk for charity

Bear in mind that activities such as those listed above have limitations in terms of team building; they likely won't be effective in addressing more serious issues such as reducing conflict or helping teams learn how to make better decisions together. In these instances, you'll want to plan a team building event with a clearly defined objective for the exercise and ensure everyone in the group participates. Facilitating a team discussion after the activity is also essential so employees have an opportunity to share feedback, their observations about teamwork and what they learned. This helps to reinforce key learnings and identify what action steps to take moving forward to enhance teamwork and engagement.

Team building activities often include some level of expense, require planning, and are more time consuming than actions to boost morale. For these reasons, most practices only schedule a few team building events each year. Be mindful to hold team building activities that promote inclusion and will be well received by all team members. It doesn't make sense to spend time and money on an event that only half the employees would enjoy or one that would make someone uncomfortable.

Managers can develop their own team building activities or seek assistance from a professional. One of the advantages of using an outside company or consultant is having an experienced facilitator for the event. Regardless of whether you work with someone else or what type of event is held, follow-up with the team is essential. Team building is not about just holding one event but rather it is an ongoing process. It can be an effective strategy to increase employee engagement if you continue to create dialogue with team members after the event about what they learned and discuss progress on agreed upon action steps.

SUMMARY

Employee retention is critical to the success of any business. Given the need for highly skilled employees and the shortage of qualified team members in veterinary medicine, it makes sense for practices to use as many strategies as possible to increase retention. It's worth noting that every chapter in this book relates to employee retention. Efforts to improve leadership, develop a positive culture, enhance team development, improve operational efficiency, and enhance profitability all contribute to increasing retention because people are more likely to stay at successful businesses with a good work environment.

In addition to paying competitive wages, the key to enhancing retention is to increase levels of engagement by increasing an employee's intrinsic rewards. Two of the best ways to accomplish this are to foster positive employee-manager relationships built on trust and to give employees some level of autonomy so they can make decisions on their own. Another is to afford team members opportunities for learning and growth. Employee development is a win-win because it helps organizations leverage the talent of employees and increases the intrinsic rewards team members feel when they gain competence and are making progress. Team building activities are also an effective employee retention strategy when they help improve team communications and create a positive work environment. Needless to say, employees are more likely to stay at a practice where everyone gets along, and the work is enjoyable.

Be aware that strategies to enhance retention may not be effective if the practice doesn't have programs in place to support the mental health and well-being of team members. Not only is team well-being important to developing a positive culture, it's critical to enhance employee retention. Team members aren't likely to stay with a practice long-term if the work environment becomes too stressful every day. This topic has been a critical focus for the profession due to high levels of stress and compassion fatigue. The need to provide programs to help support the health of veterinary teams became even more apparent when the COVID-19 pandemic gripped the nation starting in 2020. The stress of many veterinary teams worsened as a result of increased caseloads, staff shortages, operational inefficiencies related to curbside models of care and interacting with more angry clients. You can take advantage of the resources and recommendations outlined in Chapter 2 to develop and implement a comprehensive plan to enhance the team's well-being. Focusing on supporting the emotional and mental health of team members is an on-going process. Be sure to use all available resources to create effective programs and don't hesitate to seek the assistance of outside professionals.

CHAPTER 7

Communication Challenges and Solutions

The success of any practice leader hinges on their ability to communicate effectively with their team. Successful leaders clearly communicate the vision, mission, and core values of the business. They inspire and influence team members to work together to achieve practice goals. And they communicate honestly to build trust. Being an effective communicator is also a critical part of human resource management if you want to build a positive culture and enhance the team's job performance. This includes using communication skills you've learned about in earlier chapters such as how to give feedback, hold accountability meetings and manage by core values.

Constantly striving to hone communication skills is one of the characteristics of accomplished leaders. Regardless of the amount of experience you have, there is always room for improvement. Practicing the communications skills and implementing the strategies presented in previous chapters are the foundation for developing a happy, productive team. Yet despite your best efforts, you will encounter challenges with some team members. This chapter covers some of the tougher communications managers face and presents solutions to enhance your practice culture and propel your team to even higher levels of performance.

HANDLING DIFFICULT EMPLOYEES

Team members that managers either find frustrating to communicate with or who aren't performing their job as desired might be referred to as "difficult" employees. Of course, an employee one manger finds difficult may not seem difficult to another manager. Having said that, most managers find it frustrating to work with team members who aren't committed to doing a good job or don't respond positively to feedback and direction on how to improve their performance. Managers frequently say their greatest stress is dealing with employees who create drama, stir up trouble, or exhibit other types of unprofessional behavior. Team members may be viewed as "toxic" if their objectionable behavior consistently affects other employees and the culture of the practice.

Team members who exhibit difficult behaviors aren't just a problem for managers. They can significantly influence the success of the business by decreasing productivity, creating conflict with co-workers, reducing morale, and negatively affecting recruitment and retention. Moreover, difficult employees can adversely affect patient care and client care. This is why it's important to address problem behaviors as quickly as possible. Yet that doesn't always happen. Why is that?

In some instances, employees' unprofessional behavior is ignored or tolerated for months if not years. This may happen when an employee usually performs their job duties well but at times demonstrates ineffectual job performance or unacceptable behavior. Often this roller coaster of job performance occurs because an employee improves for a period of time after meeting with a manager but then gradually backslides into old patterns of behavior. Managers tend to find it hard to terminate team members who show they have the ability to do an acceptable job. Likewise, practices are reluctant to terminate an employee who is well-liked or has excellent job skills.

When confronted with addressing unprofessional behaviors, focus on two goals: helping employees improve their job performance and taking action that is in the best interest of the business. Managers must navigate deciding how much time and energy to devote to an unprofessional or underperforming employee. As with all decisions-especially those that are hard-the practice's core values serve as a roadmap. Always look to the core values and ask this question: What actions are aligned with the core values of the business? Let's say a team member has outstanding technical skills but is bullying a co-worker. To uphold the practice's core value of respect, it would be appropriate to quickly take measures to stop the unacceptable behavior even if that includes termination of employment.

It's worth mentioning the challenge managers face when they recognize the need to let go of a team member, but the practice owner or another practice leader is against termination. Perhaps the owner doctor relies on the team member's technical skills or maybe they have a sense of loyalty to them because they've worked at the practice for years. Plan to stick to factual information when discussing the employee's job performance. This is also a time to manage up; strive to get the practice owner to focus on what is best for the entire team and the success of the business.

Understanding Behavior and Managing Conversations

To help employees excel and contribute to the practice, try to understand why team members act in ways that aren't beneficial to them or the business. First, consider whether an employee's undesirable behavior is new or has been a long-standing problem. When someone has troubling actions for a long time, it's typically more challenging to change their behavior. If the problem is chronic, try to think of a time when the person didn't have the behavior as this may offer clues about what changed. Perhaps someone's job performance went downhill, for example, after an expansion of the business, or they start treating co-workers badly after a major life event such as divorce or the loss of a parent. If an employee's poor conduct is new, it's likely related to recent changes in the practice or at home which may be easier to identify.

Showing compassion and asking team members questions about their perspective can lead to greater understanding. You may uncover information you weren't aware of that could lead to turning a "difficult" employee into one with superior job performance. Perhaps you discover, for example, a veterinary assistant is exhibiting poor behavior because she is experiencing conflict with a co-worker or feels intimidated by one of the doctors. Or you may find out an employee is causing problems because they feel overwhelmed and are unhappy at work but don't feel like they have any other options but to just endure their job. To gain the most information from team members, ask multiple open-ended questions and actively listen to their responses.

Part of striving to understand employees' behavior involves being open-minded and having a mindset of genuinely wanting to help. This means approaching meetings with a team member assuming they have good intentions despite their poor performance. This is easier said than done if you're angry about an employee's disruptions or frustrated by their lack of progress. It's critical to control your emotions during employee meetings and remember to focus on the behavior, not the person. Which is why it's important to schedule a time to talk when you're calm and prepared to listen without judgement.

Asking good questions helps prevent making assumptions about why an employee chooses to act a certain way. Bear in mind questions must be non-discriminatory and appropriate for the workplace. Be sure to avoid implying job performance problems are related to race, gender, religion, sexual orientation, disability, or any other protected class. A question such as "How come I haven't seen you at church lately?" or "Are you finding it difficult to communicate with our younger employees now that you turned 50?" may seem innocuous but are actually discriminatory based on the references to religion and age. Examples of good questions are "Tell me how you're feeling about your interactions with your co-workers" and "How are you doing since we talked last time?"

During conversations with team members about their problem behavior at work, it's essential to adhere to your roles and responsibilities (and limitations) as a manager. You aren't the employee's therapist; it's imperative to focus on the needs of the business and avoid getting drawn into someone's personal problems. Be mindful to set boundaries and don't pry into an employee's personal life. Questions about an employee's health or emotional well-being could lead to unexpected and/or undesirable requests for accommodation. These questions can also encourage team members to vent about personal problems managers can't help them resolve or are better off not knowing about.

Dealing with Problem Behaviors

To develop and maintain a positive culture, confront an employee's unacceptable behavior when it occurs. If an employee lacks integrity or violates the hospital's code of conduct, you may have to terminate employment. When an employee has a lack accountability, follow the process outlined in Chapter 5 on Enhancing and Evaluating Job Performance. But in other instances, it may be less clear how to proceed. Often managers are frustrated because their attempts to eliminate bad behavior don't work. This section covers how you can confidently take action to address common problem behaviors in the workplace. Remember to document all employee conversations about job performance in the employee's personnel file regardless of whether warnings are issued.

Poor work ethic or apathy

Some team members repetitively appear to shirk certain duties or avoid work they don't like. There are several challenges when dealing with these situations. One is the employee may not always act this way, especially when practice leaders are present. In fact, they may be productive and work hard when management or the practice owner is around. Additionally, team members may diligently perform most job duties but avoid only a few job tasks they don't like. Given this inconsistency in job performance, managers may not see the problem or place a priority on addressing the issue. Another challenge occurs if the team member who displays a poor work ethic has valuable skills. A credentialed technician, for example, may want to spend all their time in surgery and post-operative patient care. They may routinely be slow to finish their work, so they don't have to complete other job duties or help with other job roles such as assisting with team training.

Apathetic employees may lack self-awareness and fail to recognize they aren't a team player. They may have a sense of entitlement especially if they have worked at the business for a long time. These team members may feel that co-workers with less tenure and experience should complete undesirable job tasks. Team members who at times avoid job tasks may be disengaged. Research shows people who tend not to pull their weight at work act this way for 3 reasons:

- The work doesn't give them intrinsic rewards (e.g., team members may find performing tasks such as dentistry procedures more valuable than helping write protocols.)
- Their contribution doesn't seem to matter or be necessary (e.g., if they wait long enough, a co-worker will do the work.)
- They don't feel a sense of belonging to the team or commitment to a common goal (e.g., rather than thinking "we're in this together", they think "why bother when I don't feel supported.")

To minimize these underlying causes of disengagement, you can emphasize the value of everyone's work contributions as a member of the team. To do this, be sure to show appreciation and recognize all employees for their individual efforts but also promote teamwork without competition.[1]

If you don't personally witness unacceptable behavior, investigate whether the complaints of co-workers are valid. This may involve talking to the veterinarians or middle managers who work with the employee. Bear in mind doctors may be unaware of the behavior especially if they like the employee and value their skills. Logically, if multiple team members complain about the work ethic of a co-worker, you may conclude the feedback is valid. But problems arise if the complaints are unfounded and borne out of jealousy and hostility. Likewise, it could be an employee with an attention to detail performs work slowly and is unfairly labeled a slacker. Therefore, the best approach is to assess the team member's overall productivity, accountability, participation in goal work, and contribution to the practice.

When it's clear someone isn't pulling their weight, talk to the employee about their job performance. This includes the veterinarians in the practice who exhibit apathy or avoid certain job duties. When speaking to team members, point out specific examples of observed behavior regarding their lack of initiative and unwillingness to do their fair share of work. Clarify (or reclarify) job expectations and make sure team members understand how co-workers perceive their inaction. Listen carefully to better understand why someone evades certain job duties or works slowly. Perhaps the employee needs more training or clarity about their job roles. If the real issue is disengagement, then put in place appropriate strategies to enhance engagement. Likewise, if the problem appears to be suboptimal motivation, focus on action steps designed to increase motivation as outlined later in this chapter.

A team member who avoids job duties needs to know specifically what they must do to improve their job performance. Depending on the severity of the problem and how long it has been going on, the best course of action may be to put in place a performance improvement plan. (See Chapter 5 on Enhancing and Evaluating Job Performance.) But if the issue hasn't been addressed previously, it may be appropriate to just outline a few actions the team member needs to take. Clearly articulate the timeline and details for requested action. Let's say a veterinary assistant avoids helping CSRs with phone calls over the lunch hour and doesn't complete job tasks at the end of their shift. The action plan might include assigning specific days and times for them to provide backup to answer phones as well as initiating a checklist of job duties they completed before leaving work. Consistently give employees feedback on their progress and provide on-going coaching since team members with a poor work ethic tend to demonstrate ups and downs in their job performance.

As much as managers would love for all employees to work well together to achieve goals and divide job duties, this doesn't always happen which is why practices should implement protocols that outline job expectations. Checklists are an excellent way to ensure team members work together to complete less desirable job duties such as keeping work areas clean, doing laundry, and completing end-of-day tasks. It may be necessary to make job assignments for items on checklists since by nature, apathetic team members find a way to avoid helping out.

Negativity

Employees who are consistently negative can be particularly aggravating for managers. They often have an endless list of items to complain about. These team members are the naysayers that find fault with everything from their co-workers, patients, and clients to how their day is going. They bring down the morale of the hospital, interfere with productivity, adversely affect client service, and create unnecessary stress for the team.

Unproductive complaining and negativity shouldn't be confused with valid employee feedback. A team member who has a reputation for being a complainer may have become critical over time because of their frustrations with poor management or other legitimate concerns. Always consider this question: "Have I listened to determine if the employee has relevant and helpful ideas or discounted them because they consistently come across negative?" If a team member does have valid concerns, they may change their behavior once they see positive change.

Sometimes employees consistently express negativity about one or more of their co-workers. This takes the form of the blame game with statements such as "I can't believe John did that-he can't do anything right", "It's not my fault we're behind schedule-Sally isn't keeping up" or "No one else around here besides me can take care of this." In these instances, help the negative team member focus on facts and accept responsibility for what they can do to help the team. Good questions to ask them include, "Is that true that John can't do anything correctly?", "How can you work with Sally and the rest of the team to stay on time?", and "How can you help with training?"

When faced with an employee who chronically complains, try to redirect their energy so it's more productive. Request that team members who bring up problems also propose solutions. If an employee criticizes workflow, for example, ask them to present ideas within one week for how to improve efficiency. This encourages people to take responsibility to affect positive change rather than just complaining. Take time to listen to team member's feedback and follow up, so they feel heard. This doesn't mean you have to implement their solution, but it does mean the idea should be given thoughtful consideration.

When employees complain relentlessly about an aspect of work that can't be changed such as safety protocols or their schedule, try to help them see how their behavior is disruptive to the work environment. Some people are naturally pessimistic and regularly come across with a negative demeanor. They don't have bad intentions and may be unaware of how their mood affects the rest of the team. Focus negative employees on the core values of the practice. If they speak negatively about clients, for example, discuss core values such as respect and compassion. Remind team members that pet owners wouldn't be in the hospital if they didn't care about their pet. Let them know that demonstrating respect and compassion for clients includes being nonjudgmental and kind.

With proper coaching, you can hopefully guide employees who always have a pessimistic outlook to adopt a more positive outlook. However, sometimes griping continues and in these situations, schedule an accountability meeting to make it clear the team member must change their behavior. Convey they have two options: They can adopt a positive mindset and focus on actions that help the team, patients, clients, and the business or they can find employment elsewhere. In these situations, it's essential to clearly communicate that continuing to be negative and disruptive is not an option.

While it isn't the job of a manager to be a counselor, it may be helpful to consider whether an employee's behavior has changed over time and whether there appears to be triggers related to their negativity. Team members with personal problems or those experiencing stress, burn-out and compassion fatigue may easily become irritable. In these cases, you can convey empathy, suggest resources for support, refer them to the hospital's EAP and encourage them to seek professional assistance.

Passive aggression

Passive aggressive behavior is defined by the Oxford dictionary as "indirect resistance to the demands of others and an avoidance of direct confrontation."[2] Passive aggressive behavior by its nature can be difficult to confront because it isn't always easy to identify. Employees who demonstrate passive aggressive behavior may indirectly indicate they will comply with job expectations but then resist with unacceptable behaviors such as gossip, blaming others, making excuses for inaction, attempting to control and manipulate others, and playing the victim.[3] (See textbox, "Examples of Passive Aggressive Behavior.")

EXAMPLES OF PASSIVE AGGRESSIVE BEHAVIOR

- Agreeing to complete job tasks but then making excuses why work wasn't completed or throwing up roadblocks for why something can't be done
- Silently refusing to train new employees and holding onto information that others would benefit from such as how to troubleshoot problems with equipment
- Refusing to give feedback or offer opinions during a team meeting and then making negative comments to co-workers after the meeting
- Pretending not to know something that was discussed or decided upon at a team meeting
- Scheduling a vacation or buying airline tickets for a trip knowing the request for time off may be denied or that the time is inconvenient for the business
- Being sarcastic towards co-workers and then saying, "I was just joking."

Managers who endeavor to understand possible reasons why employees are passive aggressive may be able to help them change their behavior. People who display passive aggressive behavior have underlying feelings and influences that cause them to act the way they do. They aren't inherently bad people. They're often angry but uncomfortable expressing this feeling. They may feel unappreciated, have low self-esteem, feel rejected or ignored, hold grudges, have a history of family problems, or suffer from anxiety and depression.[4] Since by its nature passive aggressive behavior is subtle and a covert type of behavior, you may find it helpful to remember to think about the feelings that may be associated with negative, disruptive employee actions.

When communicating with team members who exhibit passive aggressive behavior, be direct and hold them accountable for their unacceptable conduct. Focus on facts when talking about their unacceptable behavior. Let's say an employee agrees to follow a new protocol at a team meeting, but then later complains about the change or fails to follow the protocol. You can kindly confront an employee about their conflicting communications and actions with phrases such as "You indicated your support for this change during the meeting but now you aren't following our agreed upon protocol. Tell me what has changed since you agreed to follow the protocol?"

Establishing clear, agreed upon expectations and deadlines is critical when talking to a team member who appears to have passive aggressive behavior so there is no ambiguity about how they are to perform their job duties. Following the processes for how to effectively delegate and give feedback presented in Chapter 5 are essential when working with passive aggressive team members. It's wise to confirm the team member's understanding by having them repeat back to you their responsibilities or action plan. You can say "To confirm we're both clear on your action plan, can you repeat back to me your understanding of what you will do moving forward?"

Avoid becoming defensive or getting into arguments about who is to blame when talking to passive aggressive team members. Remember their underlying emotion is typically anger. Staying calm and conveying empathy work well to defuse anger. This is not to say you should get drawn into employee drama or try to fix personal problems. Simple phrases that focus on feelings are best such as "I can see you're frustrated" and "It sounds like you're feeling unappreciated." Asking open-ended questions is also beneficial to illuminate feelings and help the employee focus on facts. If a team member blames a co-worker or plays the victim, you could ask "Tell me more about your view" and "What is the evidence that Ashley doesn't like you?" The key is to help the employee understand that their feelings aren't necessarily facts. They may be making assumptions about Ashley that aren't true.

Gossip and unprofessional behavior

Perhaps one of the most pervasive objectionable behaviors in the workplace is gossip. We usually think of gossip as talking about someone behind their back. Communication exchanges involving gossip include spreading rumors, commenting on someone's personal life, and telling your co-workers about another employee's actions. Gossip could be about happy news such as "Did you hear, Linda got engaged?" Or it can be malicious such as "I found out Nancy is having an affair." Work related gossip could be a relatively innocuous comment such as "I overheard management saying we may not have our party as planned" or designed to create conflict such as "I heard Jill say that you're never willing to help her."

While it may be impossible to completely eliminate gossip, managers can inform employees what qualifies as gossip and how it can be detrimental to co-workers. When team members recognize how comments can be hurtful, they may think twice before they gossip. Encourage employees to think about their motivations before they engage co-workers in conversation that is gossip. Using the example above, what is the motivation for telling a co-worker that Jill said something negative about them? Often people gossip when they're angry, resentful, feeling unappreciated or trying to get people to choose sides. If an employee can stop and consider their feelings, they're more likely to avoid gossip and instead express their feelings. If the motivation is truly to be helpful, then the clear action would be to suggest to Jill that she talk directly to the co-worker who she feels is unwilling to help her.

Aside from creating hurt feelings and communication breakdowns, gossip damages the culture by eroding trust, decreasing morale, wasting time, and creating divisiveness.[5] Therefore, it's a good idea to create dialogue at team meetings about what constitutes gossip and how it harms the culture. Additionally provide alternative communication protocols and guidelines, so team members know what to do instead of gossiping. Here are examples of no-gossip protocols:

- No one talks about an employee who isn't present.
- Always ask yourself, "Will my comments help or hurt my co-workers?"
- If someone tries to talk to you about another employee who isn't present, decline to engage in conversation by saying "I'm not comfortable talking about _____ when he/she isn't present."
- If you overhear gossip, suggest your co-workers stop and talk directly to whoever the gossip is about.

In addition to gossip, other types of unprofessional conduct can negatively affect co-workers or the business. Unacceptable behaviors range from serious offenses such as stealing to minor offenses that some may not consider problematic. When employee behaviors are unethical, discriminatory, violate the code of conduct, or involve harassment then managers need to act swiftly to issue warnings or terminate employment. But you also want to recognize and take action to eliminate less obvious improper or undesirable behavior that disrupts the workplace and damages the practice culture.

Sometimes practices tolerate unprofessional behavior, in part, because it may fall into the category of being annoying to some people but isn't viewed as a big deal by other team members. Examples include employees who are controlling, overbearing, sarcastic, loud, messy, jokesters, or who tend to play the victim. Even if the actions are only bothersome to a few people, talk to team members who exhibit these unprofessional behaviors. Sometimes employees don't realize how they're perceived by others. Admittedly, they may not care and say, "This is just the way I am" or "I don't mean any harm." In these situations, help employees to understand how their behavior negatively affects the workplace and how it makes their co-workers feel. Then outline specific actions they must take to improve their job performance and communications.

CONFLICT RESOLUTION

Another communication challenge managers commonly face is how to handle conflict between co-workers. Some level of conflict amongst team members is inevitable and can be healthy. When conflict is minor or passes quickly, the practice culture usually doesn't suffer ill effects. But serious tension or long-standing, unresolved conflict may have damaging effects on the work environment. Therefore, it's critical that managers act as quickly as possible to resolve conflict when it occurs.

There are two basic types of conflict. Emotional conflict refers to people not getting along because of anger, resentment, personality clashes, ego, stress, or other similar feelings. With emotional conflict, team members may engage in angry discussions or arguments that are often personal in nature. By contrast, cognitive conflict, occurs when someone offers a different viewpoint or argues the merits of their ideas. Cognitive conflict can be helpful for businesses because it stimulates creativity and discussion. With cognitive conflict, team members can usually separate their personal feelings about a topic and collaborate with co-workers. It's possible for both types of conflict to occur at once. An employee may have valid concerns and merits for their position while at the same time convey emotional conflict by lashing out at a co-worker with hurtful remarks.

To identify the type of conflict, consider whether a team member is defending their position or letting their personal feelings get in the way. Emotions tend to be more intense with emotional conflict and the co-workers involved often have a history of not getting along. Emotional conflict is easier to identify when employees have personality differences or experience hurt feelings. On the other hand, if cognitive conflict occurs, team members may voice a difference of opinion but are willing to resolve their differences and move forward.

Strategies to Prevent Employee Conflict

One of the best ways to handle conflict in the workplace is to strive to create a culture that prevents conflict from becoming a problem. Managers can educate employees about communication strategies that minimize conflict and let them know what to say when it does occur. An excellent technique is to coach team members how to *respond* rather than *react* when talking to their co-workers. To illustrate the difference, have team members think of a response as maintaining control of their emotions. When people respond, they stop to think about what they want to say. By contrast, when people react, they speak quickly without regard to staying in control. Examples of reacting include sarcasm, terse comments, angry outbursts, and passive aggressive behavior. Instead of reacting, appropriate responses when conflict occurs might be "Sarah, your comments hurt my feelings. Was that your intent?" or "Kayla, I observed you didn't call Mrs. Jones as I requested. Did something come up?"

How team members handle emotionally charged situations can affect everyone's job satisfaction and set the mood for the work environment. Encourage open lines of communication between co-workers and advise them to take ownership of what they can control. Whenever possible, it's best if employees can resolve their conflict without having to involve a supervisor or manager. This helps avoid managers getting caught in the middle of a "he said, she said" scenario. When co-workers are willing to talk to each other, they may be able to resolve their differences or hurt feelings quickly. Moreover, team members who share their feelings with one another, gain a better appreciation of the other person's position and can agree to move past the disagreement. Often co-workers just need to feel like they've been heard; this helps resolve the current conflict and avoid future conflict.

To prevent conflict, be on the lookout for situations when it might become a problem. There are a variety of circumstances that are common triggers for conflict in the workplace. When new employees join the practice, they may inadvertently create conflict by talking about how they used to do things at their former place of employment. This may irritate whoever is doing their training. Conflict may occur when an employee is promoted to be a supervisor if one of their co-workers thought they deserved the position. To minimize conflict in these types of situations, make it a habit to talk to employees about job expectations and feelings they have that could lead to emotional conflict.

Facilitation of Conflict Resolution Meetings

When conflict escalates or is unresolved, it becomes a problem for both of the employees and negatively affects the success of the business. If team members can't resolve conflict on their own or feel a co-worker is unapproachable, managers may need to facilitate a conflict resolution meeting between the employees. It's not uncommon for team members who blame their co-workers for the conflict to ask managers to talk to the other employee about their concerns. This request is appropriate if the conflict involves unacceptable behavior such as harassment in which case disciplinary action would be warranted. If the conflict is long-standing or highly emotional, it may be beneficial to meet with each employee individually to gain a better understanding of their views. But ultimately, the way to successfully resolve conflict is to have employees talk to each other about their differences. (See Figure 7.1: Steps to Facilitate Conflict Resolution Meetings.)

The role of managers during conflict resolution meetings is to facilitate dialogue that helps employees understand another person's perspective and how they can collaborate to reach desired goals. Take care to remain neutral regarding emotional conflict and avoid any favoritism. And be aware of your limitations when resolving conflict. If conflict is long-standing, there are concerns about anger, or serious underlying personality problems may exist, then seek outside assistance. In these instances, it's wise to refer team members to a trained professional or the hospital's employee assistance program (EAP) for conflict resolution.

At the beginning of conflict resolution meetings, inform employees about the structure and process for the meeting, so they know what to expect. Hopefully, this information helps ease their anxiety and create a sense of safety. The next step is to concisely state the goals and purpose of the meeting. You might say "We're here today to discuss your conflict regarding job roles and assignments. During this meeting, you'll both have an opportunity to speak about your concerns and feelings. Then we'll work together to create an action plan to successfully move forward." Notice this opening also sets a positive tone for the meeting.

Prior to both employees expressing their thoughts and feelings about the conflict, establish ground rules. This includes how much time each person has to speak; ideally only two to five minutes is appropriate to avoid venting and encourage employees to be concise. Ask team members to stick to the facts and focus on observed behavior, not the other person's attitude. Additionally, instruct employees that unprofessional behavior such as name calling, raising voices and insults won't be tolerated. Lastly, request that employees listen to their co-worker and not interrupt them while they're talking. Giving each employee time to respectfully tell their story and share their feelings allows both team members to feel heard.

While listening to employees describe their view on the conflict, look for alignment so you can help both parties put aside their differences and work towards solutions to resolve the conflict. Reflective listening statements are useful to summarize the areas of alignment. You could say, "It sounds like you both have hurt feelings and feel like your views aren't respected by the other person. It's clear you both want the best for our patients and are dedicated to making that happen every day. I'm hearing that you'd like to communicate with each other in more positive ways. Does that sound right?" Once both employees have had a chance to air their grievances and articulate what they want to be different, guide them to towards an agreed upon plan for resolving the conflict.

During the process of creating a resolution action plan, anchor team members to the core values of the business; The core values serve as a roadmap to guide their actions. Rather than telling employees what they need to do, try to gain commitment by having each person propose solutions. You could say "Tell me what solutions you think would be best that are aligned with our core values." Give people time to process their thoughts if they need it or if the path forward doesn't seem obvious. You can say "I'd like you both to take the next two days to come up with specific solutions on how you can communicate and work better together that are aligned with our core values."

The written agreement should clearly state job expectations and details about the action steps both employees have agreed to take. It's wise to ask employees to focus on positive actions they want each other to take rather than focusing on negative actions to be avoided. Requesting a co-worker respectfully ask for help by saying "Could you help me?" is positive whereas saying "Stop being so critical" is negative and lacks specificity regarding what is being requested. Once employees reach agreement on the plan, set up a follow-up meeting to discuss their progress. Monitor how employees are doing and provide on-going feedback. Holding multiple meetings even when employees seem to be getting along is critical to ensure conflict truly has resolved, and team members stay focused on the goals of the business.

Table 7.1: Steps to Facilitate Conflict Resolution Meetings

Steps for Facilitators	Description
Create safety	<ul><li>Start meeting with clearly stated purpose</li><li>Outline process for meeting</li><li>Convey desired outcome of collaboration to resolve conflict</li></ul>
Encourage understanding and professional communication	<ul><li>Establish ground rules for communication:</li><li>Avoid raised voices</li><li>No accusations; only state concerns</li><li>Focus on behaviors, not attitudes</li><li>Use "I" statements, not "you" statements</li><li>Don't interrupt the person talking</li><li>Give each team member a few minutes to share their thoughts and feelings about the conflict</li></ul>
Anchor team members to the mission and core values	<ul><li>Remind team members of the common goals and mission of the business</li><li>Remind team members their behaviors need to align with the core values of the business</li></ul>
Focus on creating win-win solutions	<ul><li>Avoid favoritism</li><li>Use reflective listening statements to summarize key points of conflict and ensure team members feel heard</li><li>Look for alignment:<ul><li>What is the common ground of the co-workers?</li><li>What does each person want?</li><li>Ask team members to propose solutions</li></ul></li></ul>

Table 7.1: Steps to Facilitate Conflict Resolution Meetings (continued)

Offer assistance	• Refer team members to the business's EAP as appropriate • Suggest appropriate books, articles, videos, or blogs on conflict resolution • Give team members time to process and think about solutions if necessary

Gain commitment	• Have employees sign a written agreement
	• Define and agree on:
	  • Job expectations
	  • Specific action steps
	  • Positive communications
	  • Timeline

Monitor progress	• Give team members on-going feedback • Establish follow-up meeting(s) to discuss progress

EMPLOYEE MOTIVATION AND SELF-LEADERSHIP

A common frustration shared by managers is dealing with employees who are unproductive or seemingly lack initiative. Often these employees have excuses for their inaction. They may indicate they didn't know how to do a task or that no one was available to help them. They may suggest it was someone else's responsibility or even verbalize "That's not my job." In these instances, negativity, blaming others and decreased engagement may become part of the culture. Practice leaders are often at a loss of what to do to motivate employees who won't take ownership of their own productivity. In this section, we build on what you've learned in other chapters and outline more specific employee communications you can use to coach team members to a higher level of job performance.

Understanding Employee Motivation

Employee motivation can be defined as the amount of energy and effort people put into their work-related activities. Put another way, motivated employees are dedicated to doing a good job and have a good work ethic. To be successful, small businesses need team members to perform well and help achieve company goals. The consequences of low employee motivation include reduced engagement and productivity as well as a lack of creativity and innovation.[6] Given the importance of motivation, managers need to understand what influences employee motivation so they can focus on the best strategies to drive team performance.

Employers often assume money will motivate job performance, so they give raises and bonuses only to find positive results are short-lived, or employees still aren't motivated to excel. Giving gift cards and providing free lunches also doesn't work well to motivate employees who may develop a sense of entitlement for these rewards. Instead, the key to increasing motivation is to increase engagement. Highly engaged employees are generally motivated to do a good job because they're committed to the business and enjoy intrinsic rewards such as taking pride in their work. What this means is that managers who want to increase employee motivation need to implement strategies to increase employee engagement. (See Chapter 6 for more on employee engagement strategies.)

Sometimes practice owners or managers unfairly label an employee as someone who lacks motivation. To avoid making false assumptions, periodically meet with team members to get to know them better. The goal of these meetings is to gain a better understanding of employees' unique differences and what motivates them at work. You can accomplish this as part of a stay interview that was described in the last chapter. When meeting with employees, ask multiple questions about what they value in their job and why they want to stay at the practice. Good questions to ask include:

- "What motivates you in this job?"
- "What do you value most about your job here?"
- "What would most increase your job satisfaction?"

Asking different questions is likely to elicit a variety of responses which may be enlightening. A team member answering the first question might say they're motivated by their compensation or favorable work schedule. Team members responding to the second question may comment on how much they enjoy helping pets and people. And a response to the third question may be an expression of a desire for more training. All these questions provide insight about employee motivation. However, the first question likely speaks more about a desire for fair compensation and less about what really motivates an employee to do a good job and be engaged at work. Asking several open-ended questions provides clarity about how employees feel about their job. To fully explore a team member's motivation, an excellent follow-up question to ask is "Tell me more about that."

To improve employee motivation, think about what you're trying to achieve. Are you trying to motivate retention, accountability, improved job performance, enhanced job satisfaction, greater commitment to the business or something else? Most practice managers want to motivate enhanced job productivity and employee engagement but the strategies they use only motivate retention. The team member who receives a raise or has a schedule they like, for example, is motivated to stay in their position but may not be motivated to work harder.

Contemporary concepts on employee motivation continue to evolve. Current research shows people possess variable levels of motivation and the key to motivating employees is for leaders to guide them to optimal motivation. Susan Fowler, author of *Why Motivating People Doesn't Work...and What Does*, points out that rather than asking *if* an employee is motivated, the real question is to ask *why* they're motivated.[7] You may ask a team member, for example, why they elected to attend a continuing education event. Possible reasons might include they felt pressure or a sense of obligation, they wanted the free dinner and a chance to socialize, they were interested in the topic, or they wanted to gain new information or skills. Employees' answers help you understand their motivational outlook and level of engagement.

Fowler explains that motivation is correlated to three psychological needs people have, namely autonomy, relatedness and competency which is referred to as ARC. Her work shows that the more these needs are met, people have higher levels of motivation. Notice the similarity of these needs to the employee engagement strategies presented in Chapter 6 on Employee Retention. Autonomy is similar to empowerment; employees have some independence and can make decisions. Relatedness is the same as having purpose; employees understand the business's mission and core values as well as how they fit in. Competency is the same as employee development; employees have the skills and knowledge to do their job well.

What's perhaps most interesting about Fowler's work is her assertion that motivation is a skill that can be taught. She teaches leaders how to use three skills to obtain optimal motivation for themselves so they can in turn guide their teams to do the same. The skills are 1) to identify your motivational outlook, 2) use techniques to self-regulate your own psychological needs for ARC and 3) to reflect on the difference between suboptimal and optimal motivation. Practice managers, just like all team members, experience ups and downs in motivation. Therefore, it makes sense to understand and address your own motivational outlook so you can better guide your employees to assume responsibility for their motivation.

How To Encourage Self-Leadership

Self-leadership includes understanding one's strengths, being self-aware, setting goals, leading by example, pursuing opportunities, and taking initiative to solve problems.[8] Practice leaders should focus on their own self-leadership, not just that of employees. Being self-aware is important since this is the same quality you want to promote with team members. Begin by reflecting on your own strengths, weaknesses, and behaviors that either help or hinder you in your ability to become a successful leader. Creating a culture that encourages self-leadership leads to enhanced client service, better teamwork, higher employee engagement and increased productivity.

Effective self-leaders are positive, open to feedback, and goal oriented. They take action to help other employees and the business. They are inclined to say, "Let's do this", "We can figure this out," and "Here's what I have done." Naturally, practices tend to empower employees with these traits. However, not all employees want to be empowered and sometimes even those who are given responsibility, don't take action. Which leads to a simple definition of self-leadership that explains why even empowered team members may lack initiative. In the book *Self Leadership and the One Minute Manager*, the authors state "Empowerment is something someone gives you. Self-leadership is what you do to make it work."[9] If you have effectively empowered a team member but they still don't excel, a lack of self-leadership may be the problem.

Some empowered team members are naturally self-leaders. They always complete assignments, are happy to have additional responsibilities, take initiative to do work even during slow times, and offer solutions to problems. On the other hand, some empowered employees struggle to follow through with actions management would like them to take. This may be because they lack the additional training or communication skills needed to excel. In some instances, employees develop a victim mentality or a sense of learned helplessness. They don't think they have any power to change their circumstances, often fail to take responsibility for their job performance, and blame others for their inaction. Even talented team members can display this behavior.

Unfortunately, managers sometimes inadvertently promote learned helplessness by fostering an open-door communication policy with the team. Team members may see this as an invitation to come to the manager's office to vent about whatever they're unhappy about at the practice. Managers who listen to venting think they're being compassionate but in reality, this encourages a victim mentality. To promote self-leadership, help employees see they're not powerless and have choices. They can choose to stay stuck in a cycle of negativity and lack of accountability or they can choose to be proactive about improving their job performance and contributing to the team. (See textbox, "How to Communicate with Employees Who Have a Victim Mentality.")

HOW TO COMMUNICATE WITH EMPLOYEES WHO HAVE A VICTIM MENTALITY

- Don't give the victim a voice by offering sympathy and telling them things will be alright.
- Challenge false assumptions with questions such as "What is the evidence to support your thoughts?"
- Clearly define job roles and expectations.
- Set clear deadlines for assignments.
- Request cooperation and action with questions such as "What will you do to ensure you finish this assignment on time?" and "What will you do to be a part of positive change?"
- Insist on personal accountability.
- Provide positive feedback and recognition for excellent work.
- Ask for ideas and solutions to problems; ask "How can you help?"

One of the best ways to promote self-leadership is to empower and coach employees to be problem-solvers. This involves helping team members understand the best course of action to take when faced with challenges or difficult situations. Empowered employees do need to know their boundaries for making decisions. Remind everyone that the overarching boundary for any action is it should be consistent with the practice's mission, core values and goals. This ensures employees make decisions based on patient advocacy, excellent client service and sound business principles regarding profitability. Additionally, team members need to know specific parameters for making decisions in certain situations.

Let's look at the example of a CSR faced with an angry client who doesn't want to pay for a service on their invoice because they claim they weren't informed ahead of time about the charge. An empowered employee with self-leadership skills understands exceptional client service is a core value for the practice. They know they should take action to resolve the client dissatisfaction. But they need to know the limits for their actions. It wouldn't be reasonable to credit any amount of money on an invoice just to satisfy an unhappy client. To prepare team members to act in instances like this, they need to know boundaries such as when they can credit accounts and the limit for how much is acceptable to credit in the case of a disputed bill. Furthermore, employees need training in other ways to resolve client dissatisfaction.

To encourage self-leadership, coach team members to come to you with possible solutions, not just problems. As a starting point, ask questions to get employees to offer ideas and think on their own about how to handle challenges. Here are excellent questions to ask:

- "What have done so far to solve this problem?"
- "How do you propose we address this challenge?"
- "What ideas do you have to solve this problem?"
- "What do you think is the best course of action?"
- "What help do you need from me to solve this problem?"

Gradually, team members recognize they need to offer ideas and think about possible solutions rather than just expecting managers to fix a problem for them. With ongoing coaching, many issues that previously you had to resolve will be taken care of by the team. Bear in mind that everyone needs to understand whether they have ownership of certain job tasks. Promoting self-leadership may backfire without this clarity. A veterinary technician in charge of hospital maintenance, for example, needs to know whether they can order the repair of a piece of equipment or if they need to seek approval first for the expenditure. A fully empowered employee with self-leadership skills knows to take immediate action, who to call, how to decide on choosing the best vendor, and what to do while the equipment is out of service.

A word of caution about asking team members to be problem solvers. You may have heard (or said) the phrase, "Only come to me with solutions, not problems." This approach may discourage employees from speaking up about their challenges if they don't know how to solve a problem. Some problems are complex; an employee may not have any idea how to approach the situation or they may lack the ability to affect change. Encourage feedback and creative problem-solving but be mindful not to insist on solutions for issues that are beyond the employee's abilities or control.

Another way to encourage self-leadership is to form self-directed teams that include a small group of employees; three to six team members is ideal. Self-directed teams typically report to the practice manager or practice owner. Sometimes practices create a project team to work on specific assignments. You can use a project team to tackle hospital goals related to training, increasing compliance, improving efficiency, and improving client service just to name a few. Additionally, you can form a project team to generate creative ideas and engage in problem-solving to increase the business's success. The goal of these teams is to work together to improve hospital internal communications, identify areas for improvement, brainstorm solutions and outline specific action steps for positive change. (See Figure 7.1: Project Team Roles and Responsibilities.)

To maximize their success, self-directed teams should meet regularly to brainstorm ideas, clearly define goals, discuss how to best implement action steps to reach goals, and review their progress. The practice manager or owner act as a guide for the team; be sure to clarify the level of autonomy the project team has to avoid any misunderstandings or discord when the rest of the team. When thinking about the value of creating a self-directed team for your practice, consider these questions:

- What is the practice owner/manager doing that someone else can/should be doing?
- What systems need to be developed?
- What training needs to be done?
- What projects need to be completed?

Figure 7.1: Project Team Roles and Responsibilities

Project Team Roles and Responsibilities

Team members: _____

Oversight and direction of team: _____

Job roles and responsibilities

- Work on assigned projects and/or those identified by the project team
- Define scope of projects and suggested action plans
- Be an advocate for positive change; be a role model and cheerleader for the entire hospital team
- Solicit feedback from co-workers regarding their challenges and progress, e.g., what's working, what needs improvement, are the hospital goals clear?

Figure 7.1: Project Team Roles and Responsibilities (continued)

- Use a system to solicit employee feedback and requests, e.g., a notebook kept in central location and/or a suggestion box for staff
- Keep co-workers updated on how projects are going
- Act as liaisons for communication between departments (CSRs, technicians/assistants, DVMs, specialty services)
- Communicate with each other, other employees, and upper management in a respectful and positive manner
- Proposed solutions must meet with approval of practice manager or practice owner before implementation
- Submit requests for any required resources to practice manager or owner

Job expectations for meetings
- Meet as a team weekly or biweekly
- Schedule meetings to minimize interference with the efficiency and operations of the hospital
- Identify areas for improvement and propose solutions
- Hold each other accountable to stay positive and meet deadlines
- Draft meeting minutes (preferably typed into Word document during meetings); keep in a digital file folder and accessible notebook for reference
- Facilitate focused conversations to allow time for discussion as well as problem solving
- Establish a clear action plan with deadlines at every meeting.
- Focus efforts on a few items at a time to increase team success.
- Disseminate meeting notes to the group, manager, and practice owner after meeting

Meeting Agendas
- Review minutes and action items from previous meeting
- Review status of current projects: successes, hurdles, progress on solutions
- Review any relevant resources, e.g., articles, books, videos, etc.
- Identify projects to consider or begin work on
- Make assignments for action steps
- Set timelines and deadlines for actions
- Set date and time for next meeting

HELPING EMPLOYEES EMBRACE CHANGE

Another communication challenge you may face is trying to get team members to accept change, whether it's a new supervisor, different protocol, addition of a new service, or other changes in the workplace. People resist change for many reasons. Practice managers who take time to evaluate why their employees resist change are more likely to be successful with change management efforts. Here are common reasons team members may not embrace change:

- Fear of failure: employees might feel they can't do what is being asked of them or be afraid they can't excel with a new protocol.
- Enjoy the status quo: if team members are happy, they may not be thrilled with the need to change.
- Don't want to work harder: even team members with a good work ethic may resist change if they perceive more work will be required.
- Don't see the need for the change: team members may not understand why the change is necessary or valuable.
- Don't believe in the benefits: employees may resist change if it doesn't benefit them or there isn't a well-established benefit for patients and clients.
- Disengagement: team members may resist change because they have suboptimal motivation, or they're disgruntled.

The first step to help team members embrace change, is to remind everyone of the mission, vision, and core values of the practice. The objective is to get the team to focus on how change fits into the goals of the business. If you plan to implement a change involving client communications, for example, you may reference the practice's core value of service and how the protocol change not only helps build client loyalty but also fulfills the mission of the practice to provide outstanding patient care because it helps increase client compliance. Employees are more likely to accept change if they understand the reasoning behind the need for change.

Be honest and transparent with all communications about change. Proactively communicating details about changes and answering questions helps prevent gossip, rumors, and misinformation. You can help overcome resistance to change by giving team members a voice during feedback meetings. Not only does this alleviate fear and anxiety, but it also opens up the lines of communication. Encourage team members to express their feelings about upcoming changes and to provide feedback once change is underway. You can meet with the entire team or schedule one-on-one meetings with employees as deemed appropriate. It's essential to listen to employees in a non-defensive manner even if they criticize the need for change. Strive to validate team members' emotions, with phrases such as "I understand the changes you're experiencing may be difficult and I appreciate you sharing your concerns with me."

Focusing on words and phrases of optimism is valuable when communicating with the team. Optimists see any difficulties related to change as temporary and focus on the positive outcomes that will be a result of change. Here are some examples of optimistic messages:

- "This is temporary. We will get past these bumps in the road."
- "Right now, we're all learning this new system which can be hard. In a few weeks, it will be easier."
- "I know you're all working hard, and we are making progress towards our goal."

Inevitably someone on the team may express negativity about proposed changes. One way to deal with naysayers is to involve them in the implementation of changes. You may want to assign key responsibilities to team members who are most resistant to change. People are less critical of change if they are part of the execution process. Another way to decrease negativity is to offer employees new challenges and opportunities for growth during times of change. Such opportunities may involve new job responsibilities, continuing education, promotions, or cross-training.

For those employees who make excuses as to why they can't accept change or demonstrate passive aggressive actions, call out their unacceptable behavior. Focus on demanding honesty, transparency, and accountability. Here are some phrases to use:

- "I know you agreed in our meeting to this new protocol, but I see you aren't following it. Let's talk about why that is."
- "I observed you muttering under your breath your unhappiness with this change. Tell me what you're feeling."
- "We discussed why this change is important and what action everyone needs to take moving forward. I need for you to follow our agreed upon action plan immediately."
- "What will you do to get on-board with this change?"

It often takes time to implement changes successfully. By following the steps above, you can ease the stress associated with change and ensure a smoother transition.

SUMMARY

Team members who exhibit unprofessional behaviors or cause disruptions in the workplace can create a tremendous energy drain for managers. Everyone has a bad day occasionally but when employees consistently behave in ways that damage morale, decrease productivity and cause stress for the rest of the team, you want to act quickly to eliminate the bad behavior. Remember to assume people have good intentions and seek to understand unprofessional or troublesome employee actions. This approach is particularly helpful when facilitating conflict between team members. Hopefully, you can coach problem employees to change their unacceptable behavior and fully contribute to the practice. Using the communication skills presented in this chapter can help you guide team members to higher levels of motivation and encourage them to take ownership of their job performance.

CHAPTER 8

Hospital Operations

Hospital operations are essentially all the daily actions the business must complete to fulfill its mission and achieve goals. Operations management is the hospital system that includes activities designed to keep the practice running smoothly. Which is why when contemplating operations, we think mostly of workflow and operational efficiency. Practice managers need to routinely spend time on operational management to maximize the success of the business. Without an effective operations system, both patient care and client care may suffer as well as business profitability.

A simple definition of a system is that it is a group of processes or series of steps needed to get something done. To be successful, businesses need multiple systems. Aside from operations, the other major systems outlined in this book include financial management, marketing, client relations and human resource management. Each of these systems, in turn, needs other systems in place to accomplish goals of the system. A major goal of the human resource management system, for example, may be to develop a highly trained, productive team. To reach this goal, the practice needs effective systems for employee training and retention. Likewise, if one of the goals of your marketing system is to grow revenues, you can use multiple systems to achieve the goal. You could use the system to increase new client acquisition, improve client compliance, or recruit team members with expertise to provide more services. Each of these systems have procedures or protocols which form the processes of the system.

All hospital systems are interrelated and must function well together for the business to operate smoothly. Practices need good systems for employee recruitment and retention, for example, because the hospital can't run efficiently without sufficient staffing. Similarly, training systems work in tandem with systems involving client relations to ensure the practice can consistently deliver efficient, high quality patient care and client service. And a successful financial management system helps fund other systems in the business. Each hospital system and its supporting processes must be well established so the practice can operate smoothly even when the owner and manager aren't present. This requires planning so an evaluation of operational management should be a part of the strategic planning process outlined in Chapter 2.

In this chapter we look at specific actions you can take to improve workflow and operational efficiency as well as a few other systems not covered thus far that relate to operations. After implementing plans to improve operations, try to quantify the success of a change to see if it resulted in a positive outcome. This might include assessing daily performance measures such as client wait times and the number of client transactions as well as progress towards hospital goals. Other measures of productivity are presented in Chapter 9 on Financial Management.

OPERATIONAL EFFICIENCY

From a financial perspective, operational efficiency is about conducting business in a cost-effective, timely manner. Running a veterinary hospital is expensive and the team must deliver services efficiently for the company to be profitable. Operational efficiency is also necessary to satisfy pet owners who crave convenience and prefer practices that are easy to do business with. And veterinary teams yearn to work for practices that operate smoothly because this makes their work easier and less stressful. Simply put, the desired outcomes and benefits of enhanced operational efficiency include:

- Increased productivity: increases revenues and profitability
- Enhanced patient care: delivering efficient care means more pets can be treated
- Increased client satisfaction: convenient service results in happier, more loyal clients
- A better work environment: increases team satisfaction

To increase operational efficiency, begin by identifying signs of inefficiency. This may include:

- Consistent client wait times
- Work that doesn't get done
- Always running behind with daily caseload
- Frequent mistakes completing job duties
- No time to do client callbacks
- Breakdowns in team communication
- Missing paperwork or charts
- Items aren't in the correct location

- Team members always asking for direction
- No team member available to perform procedures or assist

Next, try to identify probable causes of inefficiency. As a starting point, it's helpful to consider if the practice has a people problem or a systems problem or both. (See Table 8.1 for an overview of the causes of inefficiency.) People problems that directly correlate with operational inefficiency include lack of teamwork, employee conflict, and employee disengagement. Action steps to address various people problems are addressed in earlier chapters.

Examples of systems problems include lack of protocols, lack of clarity on procedures or job roles, workflow issues, and ineffective scheduling. One way to decide if you have a people problem or a systems problem is to look at whether the problem involves a few employees or multiple team members. Operational systems problems typically involve multiple employees. If client wait times are a consistent problem, for example, this suggests a need to evaluate hospital processes that may contribute to inefficiency. But if only one doctor runs late, the problem likely rests with just one or two employees.

Table 8.1: Causes of Operational Inefficiency

Systems Problems	People Problems
Lack of defined policies or lack of clarity on protocols	Lack of accountability
Lack of standard operating procedures or protocols	Different doctors adhere to different standards or insist on their own way of doing procedures
Ineffective appointment scheduling	Team members don't follow scheduling protocols
Insufficient staffing	Team members unwilling to stay late or cover shifts
Workflow issues: disorganization	Lack of teamwork, employee conflict or problem behaviors, disengaged team members
Poorly defined roles & responsibilities	Lack of empowerment
Not leveraging the use of technology	Team members don't embrace use of technology or don't know to use it
Lack of training and/or skilled team members	Lack of motivation & self-leadership

Sometimes practices have both a systems problem and a people problem. For example, if the hospital has insufficient staffing this may be a systems problem if the practice doesn't have an effective recruitment system in place. But it could also be a people problem if the employee in charge of scheduling doesn't know how to create a work schedule according to the needs of the business. Likewise, a lack of trained or skilled personnel may be a systems problem if the practice doesn't have an effective training system in place but it may also be a people problem if members of the team don't have a desire to learn and grow.

Processes to Improve Efficiency

Remember a process is a set of action steps to accomplish a defined result. In medicine, clinicians follow an organized process to treat patients that starts with taking a history and doing a physical exam. Then they perform diagnostic tests to determine the best treatment plan. The same analytical approach applies to hospital operations. First evaluate what's working well and what's not working well. This includes talking to employees to gain their feedback. It may be necessary to try a new protocol to see if it will enhance efficiency. This then leads to establishing and following effective processes to reach the desired outcome of having the hospital operate smoothly. In this section, we look at common processes that influence operational efficiency.

Appointment scheduling

Challenges related to scheduling are perhaps the most common reasons cited for operational inefficiency. Figuring out how to best schedule appointments and surgeries is particularly frustrating because every hospital is somewhat different and there is not one perfect solution. Client service representatives (CSRs) tasked with scheduling have the difficult job of trying to please multiple people: practice owners who want to see a full appointment book, team members who offer opinions on how much they want scheduled, and clients that want to come in at a specific time. CSRs also routinely make appointments for patients with medical conditions they have limited knowledge about so they may not always schedule these patients according to the desires of various team members. In addition to providing sufficient training for the front office team, try to evaluate other ways to modify the process of scheduling to improve operational efficiency.

When evaluating scheduling, start by looking at the capacity of the appointment book. Are all the doctors fully booked each day or week or do they routinely have several open appointment slots? How quickly does the appointment schedule fill up? How long does it take for clients to get in for appointments after they call the practice? Is there a long wait time for patients needing routine surgeries or dentistry? Has the practice had to limit the number of new clients or is there a waiting list for new clients who want an appointment? This assessment can help determine whether operational inefficiencies are related to the practice being at full capacity or due to other challenges such as staff shortages and lack of training.

Next, look at the time allotment for appointments. Most general practices book 20-30 minutes for appointments and specialists typically book up to an hour. Hospitals that only book 15-20 minutes for all appointments tend to have more problems with efficiency. It's simply not practical or reasonable to expect veterinarians to perform a physical exam, thoroughly educate clients about the value of services and treat sick patients efficiently if they have short appointment times. And when doctors have back-to-back appointments with sick pets or those with multiple conditions, this situation magnifies problems with operational efficiency. The solution in these instances is to allow more time for appointments even if this means fewer appointments each day. Some practice owners are reluctant to decrease the number of appointments because they fear a loss of revenue. This is short-sighted thinking because giving doctors longer appointments affords them more time to talk to clients. Increases in client satisfaction and compliance combined with other measures such as increasing day admissions can easily lead to greater revenues rather than a loss of income.

Busy practices need to block appointments for same-day sick patients or emergencies. Deciding how many appointment slots to block each day depends on the number of doctors and the caseload. Some hospitals only need one or two appointments each day while others may need to block multiple appointments to ensure sick patients can be seen in a timely manner. It's not unusual for veterinarians-especially practice owners-to double book appointments. While this facilitates fitting in more patients, the long-term effects can be detrimental to the practice. Negative consequences include compromised patient care, decreased client satisfaction due to wait times, breakdowns in communications, poor client education, and increased team burnout.

Another way to improve operational efficiency is to see if you can create more appointment slots each week. Rather than double booking, the practice might be able to increase capacity by adding appointments earlier in the morning or later in the day. If the first appointment of the day is currently at 9am, perhaps you can add an appointment at 8:30am. For practices with multiple doctors, you can stagger the doctor's lunch breaks and this may allow you to add an appointment slot during the lunch time. Increasing day admissions of patients is another way to see more patients. Doctors can see these pets in between appointments or before the lunch period. Remember that while these strategies may increase capacity and efficiency, the practice has to have a sufficient number of team members to handle the increased caseload.

Practices may be able to increase productivity and efficiency by scheduling technician appointments for services that don't require a doctor such as nail trims and second booster vaccinations. Technician appointments are helpful because they free the veterinarians up to see more pressing cases. Bear in mind that for this strategy to work well, the hospital must have sufficient staff to take care of the extra technician appointments and mangers need to assign roles so it's clear which team members will see these patients.

Patient admission and discharge

Evaluating the hospital's patient admission and discharge process is another effective way to improve operational efficiency. Because multiple clients tend to arrive all at once, these times often create bottlenecks for the team. Moreover, clients dropping off or picking up their pets don't like to wait and can quickly become irritated. Efforts to streamline these processes lead to greater efficiency and client satisfaction. Giving clients a specific appointment time to drop off and pick up their pet can help increase efficiency. This solution isn't perfect because inevitably some clients will still arrive at the same time especially when dropping off patients in the morning. Scheduling appointments for afternoon patient discharges, however, tends to work well because people typically aren't in a hurry to get to work or take children to school.

An essential step to include as part of the admission and discharge process is to clearly define the flow of communication between CSRs and members of the technical team. When the front office team doesn't know who's in charge of admitting and discharging patients or they have to track down a team member, this wastes time. Managers can collaborate with veterinary technicians and assistants to create a defined, written admission and discharge process that saves time while still delivering quality patient and client care. The process might include:

- Usage of online client information forms
- Staggered client appointment times every 15 minutes
- Preparing patient files prior to client arrival
- Designating the employee(s) each day who will admit/discharge patients

- Using a checklist to ensure team members secure appropriate information for admissions
- Using a form to give clients written patient discharge instructions

Exam room flow

One of the most neglected, yet critical processes that directly affects operational efficiency is exam room workflow. Organized teams can minimize client wait times and see more patients. To improve appointment efficiency, start by clearly defining team member's roles and responsibilities. Designate specific employees to assist in exam rooms each shift. Otherwise, assisting in exam rooms becomes a free-for-all and it's easy for team members to get caught up in other duties or avoid helping in rooms. Many hospitals find it works well to assign specific team members to work with each veterinarian, so the doctors know who will assist them with appointments each day.

It's helpful to post assigned job roles in a visible location for the entire team to be able to see who will handle specific job duties each day. This includes which employees will draw blood samples and perform diagnostics for patients in exam rooms, who will fill medications, and who doctors should ask when they need more help. Furthermore, it's helpful if hospital teams clarify who will review treatment plans with clients and who will educate clients on topics related to preventive care and home care instructions. Without defined job responsibilities, work can seem chaotic. Not only is operational efficiency a problem in these situations, but managers may face difficulties with employee accountability.

Another strategy to improve exam room workflow is to establish specific procedures that help employees stay organized and save time. Implementing multiple action steps can add up to significant improvements in operational efficiency. For example, using some type of flag system outside exam room doors helps everyone know the status of rooms-whether it's occupied, available for use, ready for a specific doctor, needs cleaning, etc. Making sure charts, check-in sheets, lab results or travel sheets have a designated home helps with efficiency, so people don't waste time trying to find paperwork. Likewise, stocking exam rooms with all the necessary supplies and equipment saves time because team members don't have to leave the room to retrieve something. Avoiding taking pets in and out of rooms also increases efficiency because it eliminates the time it takes employees to relocate patients. Performing simple diagnostics and treatments in exam rooms saves time and is consistent with Fear Free® techniques that minimize stress for pets.

Leveraging technology

There are multiple ways practices can use technology to enhance exam room efficiency. When pet owners fill out client information forms prior to their appointment, this saves time during check-in and in exam rooms. Typically, technicians or assistants gather a patient history from clients in the exam room. Doctors frequently complain if team members spend too much time taking a history because it can delay them starting their appointment. An easy way to obtain a more detailed history and improve efficiency is to have clients fill out a history form online. Then team members can review the information and concentrate on asking specific, relevant questions related to the pet's reason for coming in.

Another effective use of technology is to have prepared treatment plans for common medical treatments, dentistry procedures, and surgeries so team members don't have to generate a new treatment plan for every client. Managers can use the practice management software to link service codes for services that are typically done together when creating treatment plans. Another action step that saves time is to reduce the number of computer codes for services because this creates confusion when employees look up the cost of services or seek to add items to an invoice. It's frustrating and inefficient having to stop and ask a co-worker or the doctor which code to use.[1]

Implementing Protocols and Standard Operating Procedures

Hospital processes usually work better when team members follow specific protocols and procedures when completing work. The terms protocol and standard operating procedure (SOP) may be synonymous depending on how they're used. However, the difference is that a protocol usually refers to a rule (or set of rules) while an SOP refers to the method for completing a job task. Examples of protocols include radiation safety protocols, surgical site preparation protocols, vaccine protocols, and isolation room cleaning protocols. Examples of SOPs include methods for patient admissions, filling prescription refill requests, exam room client communications to increase compliance, and performing a comprehensive physical exam on a patient.

Protocols may be part of a SOP. For example, when taking radiographs, one of the protocols is that employees must wear protective gowns and gloves. This safety protocol is part of the SOP for taking radiographs which includes the steps employees follow to get the desired views of the patient. When drafting protocols and SOPs, include the rationale for the procedure as well as any relevant details about how to complete it. (See Figure 8.1: Protocol Template and Figure 8.2: SOP Template.) From a practical standpoint, you can use the template that makes the most sense and provides clarity for team members. Use bullet points when outlining the details of a procedure to make documents easier to read.

Figure 8.1: Protocol Template

PROTOCOL TEMPLATE

When drafting protocols, include the following as appropriate:

1. **Purpose:** (Why does the protocol exist; why is it important)
2. **Roles/Responsibilities:** (Outline team member job roles; who can perform duties and when)
3. **Details of protocol:** (Outline specific steps that must be taken and/or relevant details about how the protocol must be followed)

Figure 8.2: SOP Template

SOP TEMPLATE

When drafting a standard operating procedure (SOP) include the following as appropriate:

1. **Purpose** (What is the goal of the procedure; why is it important)
2. **Summary** (Summarize the procedure and expectations for how it should be performed)
3. **Definitions** (Explain any terminology or abbreviations, as necessary)
4. **Qualifications/Responsibilities** (Outline the qualification required of the person who can carry out the procedure and a general description of the responsibilities involved)
5. **Procedure** (Provides in detail the step-by-step instructions to complete the procedure)

Establishing protocols and SOPs

The primary reason for establishing protocols and SOPs is to maintain the desired quality of patient care and client care. Implementing standard procedures helps provide clarity within the organization so everyone consistently completes job tasks according to established standards. Moreover, when team members know how they're supposed to perform job duties, this saves time.

If you're a manager faced with putting into place a substantial number of practice protocols and SOPs, this may seem like a daunting challenge. To successfully complete this project, you'll want to enlist assistance from your team. To begin, look at hospital operations and have team members help create a list of practice protocols and procedures. The list may include well-established procedures that everyone knows as well as ones that are missing or unclear. Most practices, for example, have clear vaccine protocols but lack SOPs in areas of operations such as appointment scheduling, equipment maintenance, client communications, and exam room workflow. Additionally, solicit feedback from team members with these questions:

- Is the protocol or procedure clear?
- What details are missing?
- Is the protocol or SOP in writing?
- Do team members know where to read the protocols and SOPs?
- What protocols does the practice need to develop?
- What SOPs does the practice need to develop?
- Does the practice have protocols or SOPs that team members aren't following?

You can create a list of procedures and gain feedback for the above questions by holding a brainstorming session during a team meeting. Alternatively, you can post large pieces of paper from a flip chart on a wall in the hospital so employees can write down information about protocols and SOPs during the workweek.

Once you have a complete list of practice protocols and SOPs, the next step is to organize your list. You may want to arrange each item under one of three headings according to whether it is 1) clear and already written, 2) clear and just needs to be drafted, or 3) needs to be clearly defined and then put in writing. Since managers aren't always familiar with all practice procedures, it's important to have team members who are responsible for following the procedures be involved in writing the practice's protocols and SOPs.

You can then group written documents into categories for easy reference by team members. File electronic documents in folders on all computer workstations and put a notebook with the printed protocols and SOPs in a central location in the hospital so team members can easily access the information. Here are a few examples of categories:

- Safety protocols
- Hospital cleaning protocols
- Outpatient medical procedures
- Surgery room and anesthesia monitoring
- Exam room protocols
- Client communications
- Appointment scheduling
- Patient Admission and Discharge

When developing protocols and SOPs, prioritize drafting the most important ones first. You want to clarify and establish procedures related to patient care, for example, before spending time on developing a protocol for how to submit a lab request for a test that doctors rarely order. Likewise, focus first on protocols and SOPs that involve the most patients and clients. An example is protocols for exam room client communications.

Another way to think about the prioritization of drafting protocols and SOPs is to consider pain points for both clients and the team. What do people complain about most often? When and why do clients have to wait? What are frequent questions employees ask about how to do their jobs? When do breakdowns in communication or errors occur? It makes sense to focus first on establishing SOPs that are the most desirable to increase operational efficiency and client satisfaction.

One pitfall to be aware of occurs when practices implement a protocol that favors the team, but pet owners don't like it. An example is requiring 24-hour or more notice for a prescription refill request. The protocol is designed to give doctors time to review medical charts and approve the request. The problem for clients is that most of them are used to getting their prescriptions faster from human pharmacies and they may have a sense of urgency if they're out of medication. To address this challenge, you could create a new SOP that includes setting up client reminders for medication refills, appointing specific team members each day to refill medications, and blocking time for doctors to review refill requests so the team can process requests quicker.

But what happens if team members don't follow established procedures? The key is to ascertain why someone isn't complying. Sometimes the problem stems from a lack of clarity or training. SOPs shouldn't be so complicated as to be difficult to read and learn (unless they're medical in nature). To avoid this scenario, prior to rolling out SOPs or new protocols, hold team meetings to give employees an opportunity to ask questions. These meetings also help team members understand the importance of following procedures. And lastly, continue to check in with team members about the hospital's procedures. You can ask, "What's working well with this protocol?", "What still needs clarity?", and "How can we improve training?"

Setting medical standards

Medical standards define details about patient treatments and the level of care. Examples of medical standards include vaccine protocols, sterilization procedures, preventive care guidelines, sanitation and disease control standards, pre-anesthetic testing protocols, and pain management protocols just to name a few. Setting hospital medical standards helps ensure the consistency, quality, and continuity of patient care. As with operational SOPs and protocols, medical standards also help increase efficiency because everyone knows what to do which keeps the practice running smoothly.

Standards such as puppy vaccine protocols and the SOP for surgical site preparation for sterile surgery are well known procedures presumably followed by all practices. But most practices still lack clear medical standards in many areas. A survey conducted by the Veterinary Hospital Manager's Association found that fewer than 50% of the practices surveyed had standards in place for pain management, nutritional recommendations, and laboratory testing.[2] Other examples where hospitals tend to lack standards of care relate to patient diagnostics and medical treatments. If a dog presents for otitis externa, for example, do all your doctors recommend an otic cytology? Is it a standard to recommend and forward book medical progress exams for pets with certain conditions? Does the hospital follow recommended industry guidelines for fecal and heartworm testing? When standards aren't clear, employees have to ask for direction and workflow slows down.

To establish medical standards, managers must work with the veterinarians in the practice to reach consensus. The goal is to get doctors to agree on standards that align with the core values of the practice and medical guidelines. For example, all doctors should be able to agree on the hospital standard for pre-anesthetic laboratory testing of pets and the need for annual heartworm testing. In some instances, standards may not be clearly dictated by medical experts. Veterinarians don't like to be told how to practice and at times will need the flexibility to respond to difficult situations such as when pet owners have limited funds, or a pet is near end of life.

HOLDING EFFECTIVE TEAM MEETINGS

For practices to run smoothly, team members need to understand hospital protocols, communicate effectively with each other, and work well together. One of the best ways to promote teamwork and excellent communication is to hold successful team meetings. For a team meeting to be successful, it needs to be productive which can be easier said than done. Even experienced managers have the challenge of making sure meetings don't turn into gripe sessions. Likewise, managers may have to deal with employees who don't find value in meetings or refuse to participate. Another widespread problem is discovering that a meeting didn't lead to anticipated positive change, or the change is short-lived.

Define The Purpose and Agenda of Meetings

The first fundamental element for success, is to make sure every meeting has a clear purpose. Team meetings are an excellent time to disseminate information, discuss hospital operations, provide training, brainstorm new ideas, and facilitate problem solving. Gaining clarity and focus before the meeting helps you stay on track and run a more efficient meeting. Consider the answer to these questions before scheduling each meeting:

- What is my desired outcome?
- What question needs to be answered?
- What problem do we have?
- What solution do we need?
- What information must we share?
- What type of team training do we need?

No one wants to be in a meeting where the topic of discussion isn't relevant for them so always consider who benefits from the meeting. A meeting to review anesthetic protocols or laboratory equipment, for example, may not be pertinent for client service representatives. In this instance, it may be better to schedule a meeting just with the technicians and assistants involved with surgery and lab testing. Additionally, holding smaller, departmental meetings is often more effective than larger meetings because a small group can discuss a topic and brainstorm solutions more quickly.

Sometimes practice owners and managers express their frustrations about lack of accountability during team meetings thinking this will get everyone on track. Managers might, for example, remind everyone to get weights on all pets admitted to the hospital, complete all call backs as assigned, or remember to forward book appointments. If a problem with an operational process or protocol involves the entire team, then it's valuable to discuss the topic, gain feedback and engage in problem-solving. But in instances where the lack of accountability only involves a few people, it's counterproductive to address the issue in a team meeting. Usually, those employees with poor job performance don't take the message to heart and the rest of the team is frustrated listening to admonishments that don't apply to them. Rather than taking up time at a team meeting, schedule an individual accountability meeting to discuss job performance issues with employees.

Another best practice is to plan the meeting agenda ahead of time and post it prior to the meeting, so employees know what to expect. Whenever possible, afford team members the opportunity to submit ideas or requests for the agenda by a specific deadline. It's then up to the meeting facilitator or practice manager to decide whether to include the subject for discussion on the agenda. When reviewing requests, decide whether a topic is appropriate for the team meeting. If you can't include an employee's idea on the agenda, let the team member know why their topic isn't relevant or is being deferred to a later time. Given the time constraints of team meetings, it's important to prioritize agenda items. One way to save time is to consider whether announcements benefit from face-to-face communication or if you could easily convey the information in a written memo distributed via email or a messaging app.

Regardless of the purpose of a meeting, it's ideal to start all-team meetings with 5-10 minutes of positive feedback and success stories. Recognition and praise can come from the practice owner, managers, or co-workers. Many practices have a system to collect written appreciation from team members who notice when a co-worker works hard or is especially helpful. The positive feedback is then shared at the next team meeting. If you have rewards such as gift cards tied to whoever gets the most accolades, just be sure the team feels the system is fair and enjoyable.

The Art of Facilitation

Meetings may be ineffective if the person running the meeting lacks good facilitation skills. Therefore, whoever is in charge of leading any part or all of the meeting needs to understand aspects of effective facilitation. The choice of meeting facilitator is often based on the nature of the meeting and topics for discussion. The practice owner may be the preferred facilitator if one of the goals of the meeting is to review major changes in hospital policies or compensation packages, since they'll be able to answer questions and provide the reasoning behind the changes. Generally speaking, practice managers facilitate all-team meetings and supervisors, or team leaders facilitate smaller departmental meetings. Some hospitals like to rotate different employees each month as the facilitator. This can work well to promote leadership skills as long as managers provide coaching for team members in the art of facilitation. (See Figure 8.3: Job Description for Meeting Facilitators.)

The practice manager or facilitator should assign a team member to keep notes during the meeting. This is because it's difficult to effectively facilitate and take notes at the same time. The role of the note-taker is to capture key points from discussions for the meeting minutes. Meeting scribes can use a tablet or laptop during the meeting and type notes into a template so all they have to do is add bullet points about relevant information. The facilitator or manager can then review the minutes for accuracy and post or email the notes to all team members after the meeting. Team meeting notes should also be filed electronically and placed in an accessible notebook for easy review/reference.

Set Deadlines and Establish Action Plans

Even when lively and productive discussion occurs during team meetings, outcomes may be minimal or non-existent if an action plan isn't put in place. Action plans need to detail work assignments regarding *who* will act and *when*. Bear in mind deadlines for action items don't have to be the date of the next meeting. It's more efficient to set an earlier deadline for team members to work on assignments and report to the manager upon completion. This facilitates more progress towards achieving goals between meetings. For positive change to occur, try to avoid ending meetings with phrases such as "we need to do a better job of…." or "let's all remember to do…." While everyone may agree with the sentiment, nothing is likely to change if managers don't outline specific actions that will lead to different behaviors and outcomes.

Figure 8.3: Job Description for Meeting Facilitators

Job Description for Meeting Facilitators

Team meeting facilitators are responsible for leading the team through the meeting agenda. Facilitators are expected to be energetic, remain neutral, actively listen, and advocate for positive change.

The roles of the facilitator include the following:

- Start and end meetings on time.
- Start each meeting by reviewing the action items from the last meeting.
- Adhere to the agenda. Be cognizant of time limits for the meeting and keep discussion moving. If there are 3 topics, the facilitator may break up the meeting into 3 segments of time to keep the group on track.
- Encourage and request participation from the group. Facilitators ask for feedback from the rest of the team rather than spending a significant amount of time talking.
- Facilitate effective dialogue. Every employee doesn't need to talk at every meeting. But facilitators should avoid having the same few people monopolize the conversation while other employees remain silent.
- Ask questions to stimulate creativity, conversation, and feedback.
- Encourage problem-solving. Avoid using phrases such as "we need to talk about" and instead use meaningful action verbs such as "coordinate, brainstorm solutions, share ideas, create plans, and solve problems."
- Before initiating discussion, have team members take 5 minutes to write down their ideas on paper. This encourages individual creativity, ensures participation by everyone, and may help introverted individuals give feedback. Employees then take turns sharing what they wrote down.
- Summarize employees' responses into main themes or agreed upon ideas. Use reflective listening statements such as, "It sounds like everyone agrees on...." or "It appears everyone feels ____ is a problem that needs to be addressed."
- Remain calm during heated discussions. Attempt to resolve conflict by validating the feelings of participants and looking for ways to create win-win scenarios for the team.
- Keep the team focused on the topic. When employees focus on peripheral issues or start rehashing discussion topics, facilitators need to get everyone back on track.
- Stay positive and re-direct unproductive or negative dialogue.
- Work with the team to establish clear action plans, assignments, and timelines.

Standing Meetings and Morning Huddles

Medical rounds are the classic standing meetings all doctors are familiar with. During these meeting, doctors present a patient case to other doctors during training programs or review patient care instructions at shift changes in larger hospitals. Practices can use short standing meetings for multiple other reasons. Many hospital teams like to conduct morning huddles to share relevant news and review the day's appointments. Standing meetings also work well to conduct brief training sessions, share success stories, debrief at the end of a day, convey important announcements, and discuss progress on a new initiative. Standing meetings are typically 5-15 minutes in length.

For morning huddles, decide who will keep the meeting on track. This could be an associate doctor, manager, team leader or practice owner. You may decide to rotate this role at your practice. Daily huddles can help improve internal communications and enhance operational efficiency. They aren't meant to be used for problem-solving or in lieu of regular staff meetings. Meetings should start and end on time. Be sure to include at least one representative from all departments. Here are ideal topics for these meetings:

- Review the day's schedule, workflow, and role assignments
- Convey alerts-e.g., euthanasia, new clients, difficult clients, or aggressive pets
- Review client care preferences
- Quick announcements or reminders
- Acknowledgments-e.g., birthdays, anniversary, accomplishments
- Focus on core values
- Share quick success stories

INVENTORY MANAGEMENT

To operate smoothly, hospitals must have a suitable inventory of drugs and supplies on-hand for all procedures, treatments, surgery, and take-home medications for patients. When practices run out of something, employees and managers must spend time figuring out how to solve the problem which reduces efficiency and productivity for the hospital. However, you want to keep quantities on hand to a minimum given the tremendous cost of inventory. As discussed in Chapter 9 on Financial Management, the cost of goods sold is one of the greatest expenses for a practice. Therefore, effective inventory management is critical to profitability as well as operational efficiency.

This section includes a brief overview about how to improve the efficiency of inventory management. Managers that want more information on inventory management should consult additional resources and take advantage of training opportunities to learn more. Dr. Marsha Heinke's book, *Practice Made Perfect*, available from AAHA has a chapter devoted to inventory control and management. Multiple veterinary magazines, associations, and companies also routinely publish articles on inventory management.

Designate an Inventory Manager

Practice managers should clearly define the job roles, responsibilities, and expectations for any team member involved in inventory management. Most practices assign a technician or assistant to place inventory orders since they're familiar with hospital drugs and medical supplies. Often other employees share the responsibility to create order lists, unpack boxes, process invoices, update prices in the practice information management software (PIMS), place special orders, and oversee the hospital's online pharmacy. The difficulties that can arise with this approach of having multiple team members complete job tasks are breakdowns in communication and poor inventory management.

To avoid these problems, its ideal to designate an inventory manager who is in charge of inventory management and control. Inventory managers need to be detail-oriented, well-trained, and dedicated to saving the practice money. To maximize the effectiveness of inventory managers, practices are wise to invest in providing them training opportunities. Multiple companies and associations offer courses on inventory control and management.

Large hospitals may have a full-time inventory manager, but most practices have someone in this position whose primary job role is as a member of the technical team. In these situations, the person in charge of inventory needs a schedule that includes blocks of uninterrupted time to complete their inventory job duties. Depending on the size of the practice, inventory management can be time-consuming. It's reasonable to have other employees assist with specific job tasks, but the inventory manager needs to maintain oversight and coordinate with the practice manager to ensure the practice has a cost-effective and efficient inventory management system.

It's not uncommon for practices to implement a protocol of having employees write a product on a list or tell the manager when inventory items are low. This process is inefficient and commonly leads to higher inventory expenses. Instead, hospitals should strive to use the PIMS to track and manage inventory. Most software companies have representatives or courses that provide specific training, so managers know how to take advantage of all the benefits of their program. Regardless of whether the practice uses the PIMS or a manual system to track inventory, inventory managers should allocate specific, defined hours to inventory management each week and establish set days to place orders (ideally online) rather than placing orders every day as needed. This improves operational efficiency and ensures there are enough drugs and supplies on the shelf without overstocking products.

Determine Quantity on Hand and Reorder Points

Quantity on hand is defined as the amount of an inventory item to stock so the hospital has sufficient drugs and supplies prior to the next order. To establish minimum quantity on-hand amounts, determine how much of an item needs to be on the shelf, so the hospital doesn't run out of supplies but also factor in not having excess inventory. For practices that receive inventory orders from major distributors within a few days from the time they're ordered, it's usually safe to only stock the amount of product to last 10 to 14 days. Be sure to account for approximate shipping times and dates of delivery for inventory items when deciding on quantity on hand amounts.

Since it's hard to predict exactly how much inventory the practice will use each week, look at the quantity of medications and supplies used in a one to two-month period as a starting point. You may need to adjust the quantity on hand amounts seasonally or prior to known peak times. During the summer months, for example, a general practice may need to stock more flea and tick preventives and prior to holiday weekends an emergency hospital may need to stock up on fluids and other commonly used drugs.

To minimize overstocking and keep costs down, strive to turnover inventory quickly so it isn't sitting on the shelf for long. The rate of inventory turnover refers to the number of times inventory is used and replaced in one year's time. The ideal inventory turnover is eight to twelve times per year. Managers can run PIMS reports that detail the monthly usage of drugs and supplies. If they notice products stay on the shelf longer than 4-6 weeks, this signals an opportunity to reduce inventory and spending. Additionally, managers can request ABC usage reports from distributors that show which drugs and supplies the business orders most often. Items in the "A" category may need to be stocked in higher quantities due to frequent usage and it may be more cost effective to eliminate a "C" item or move it to the hospital's online pharmacy to reduce costs.

Set up re-order points for all inventory so it's clear when to place the next order for the product. The purpose of the re-order point is to know when to restock drugs and supplies before there is a significant risk that the hospital might run out of the item before it receives the next order. Let's say for example, your hospital has a quantity on hand amount for 5mg Prednisone of two bottles. You might establish a re-order point to purchase another bottle once your quantity on hand is down to one bottle. It can be difficult to know the ideal re-order point since you don't know exactly how long it will take to consume or sell inventory items. For commonly used items such as fluids and antibiotics, re-order points are generally set to maintain a greater quantity on hand than for less commonly used items. Establishing re-order points for each inventory item is time-consuming but well worth the time spent to improve efficiency and cost-savings long-term.

Inventory managers should coordinate with the practice manager or owner to keep inventory costs in line with established budgets and industry benchmarks. One way to do this is to create a weekly Inventory budget based on a target goal for the cost of goods sold as a percentage of revenues. For drugs and supplies, the target goal might be 15-19% of gross revenues. If you factor in all variable expenses such as lab expenses and imaging costs, then the goal may be 23-25%. To set the budget each week, managers can look at the gross revenues from the previous week. [Example: the previous week's gross revenue multiplied by target goal: $28,000 x 20% = $5,600 maximum to spend the next week]. Managers should be careful to avoid too many deals and promotions unless they are confident the practice will use and sell the drugs and products quickly.

It's important to establish appropriate price markups in the PIMS for all inventory items. Commonly reported target markups for most drugs range from 140-175 percent of the cost of the medication including sales tax and shipping. The target markup for flea, tick and heartworm preventives is usually less so the price of these products is competitive with other sellers. Due to competition from online pharmacies, some practices reduce their markups for select products closer to a 50 percent markup.

Remember when pricing inventory items, to consider all the costs associated with selling the product and the desired profit margin. You also want to evaluate the practice's pricing strategy and level of competition when deciding how to mark-up products. Again, seeking added training on this topic is beneficial for both practice managers and inventory managers. Lastly, don't forget to always enter price updates in the PIMS when the cost of drugs and supplies increases.

Summary

For a practice to operate efficiently, it needs a system of clearly defined processes and procedures, so team members know how to complete their work and stay organized. Operational efficiency (or lack thereof) affects patient care, client care, employee engagement and profitability. Therefore, it's critical to spend time evaluating operations so you can implement missing protocols, create SOPs, and enhance processes that lead to greater efficiency and productivity. Of course, people run operations so facilitating effective team meetings is paramount to the success of any practice. Often the best ideas to improve operations come from employees. Lastly, every practice needs an effective inventory management system which helps to keep the hospital running smoothly and saves the business money.

CHAPTER 9

Financial Management

Financial management includes all the activities business stakeholders take to plan, organize, oversee, and control the financial resources of the business. Effective financial management is critical to the long-term success of any practice. Without good financial management, the business may not make a profit and thus fail. Solid financial management is also imperative to make sure there are sufficient funds to achieve business goals related to other areas of the practice such as patient care, operations, team development, culture, client relations and marketing. To ensure the long-term success of the business, practice owners should maintain oversight of all aspects of financial management.

Practice managers play an integral role in ensuring the financial health and profitability of the business. How much responsibility managers assume for financial management varies depending on their job description, the ownership of the practice, and the roles that other professionals such as accountants and bookkeepers have in the business. For some practices, the hospital administrator or practice manager might create budgets, manage cash flow, maintain major practice expense categories within target goals, make purchasing decisions, work directly with the accountant and be accountable to the business owner for successfully completing these job duties.

On the other end of the spectrum are managers with minimal to no financial management duties. Regardless of their job description, all managers need to have a clear understanding of what factors affect profitability as well as the relationship between the financial position of the practice and other areas of management such as team development. For example, it's helpful for managers to know payroll expenses when making decisions about employee recruitment and pay increases. Likewise, managers who want to analyze team productivity need to understand data related to practice revenues and staff to doctor ratios. In this chapter, we look at the most important aspects of financial management mangers should know about even if they don't have direct responsibility in that area.

KEY PERFORMANCE INDICATORS

Key performance indicators, or KPIs, are defined as a quantifiable measure used to evaluate the success of an organization or individual in meeting objectives for performance.[1] An assessment of these metrics reveals how the business compares to similar businesses and how well the company is doing in meeting its goals. In veterinary medicine, the most common KPIs practices should track are related to revenues, doctor productivity and client data. Evaluating KPIs helps practice owners and managers decide if they need to make changes to improve financial health and profitability.

KPIs are useful because they provide specific information about different aspects of the business. An evaluation of multiple KPIs tells a story about the financial well-being of the business. You can review most of your practice's KPIs, especially those related to revenues, by running reports in your Practice Information Management System (PIMS). KPIs for expenses come from accounting software reports. In this section, we review important key performance indicators every practice should routinely monitor and why. To learn more about the actual numbers reported for various KPIs you can reference other sources that publish veterinary practice data.

Industry Benchmarks

The terms "industry averages", "standards" and "benchmarks" are often used interchangeably which can be confusing. The Merriam-Webster dictionary defines a benchmark as "something that serves as a standard by which others may be measured or judged."[2] Since benchmarks are essentially desired standards, they serve as target goals. On the other hand, industry averages refer to the average number for a database. This number may or may not be a desirable target goal. When looking at data for the veterinary profession, look at the sample size of the database and details about the businesses included in the survey. Ideally, you want to compare your practice data to data from similar practices. Moreover, it's beneficial to know benchmarks for profitable practices and then compare your KPIs to businesses in that database.

Several associations and organizations publish financial data for the veterinary industry. This includes Well-Managed Practice® Benchmarks which reports data each year for 100 successful veterinary practices that must meet criteria before being included in the benchmark study. The American Animal Hospital Association (AAHA) publishes practice statistics usually every 2 years. Its vital statistics series includes Financial and Productivity Pulsepoints, Compensation and Benefits and the Veterinary Fee Reference. The Veterinary Hospital Managers Association (VHMA) reports monthly on a few key economic indicators of how its member practices are performing with respect to revenue growth, the number of patient visits and the number of new clients. The organization also publish a bi-annual compensation and benefits survey report for its members.

In 2020, the American Veterinary Medical Association (AVMA) partnered with the company VetSuccess to provide revenue and compliance data for the profession with a tool called the Veterinary Industry Tracker. This tool collects data from thousands of practices and compares KPIs from the current year to the prior year. Other organizations such as corporate veterinary practice groups and Veterinary Study Groups (VSG) compile data for their member hospitals and generally only provide financial reports to practice owners and managers in the group.

You can also read numerous articles and other publications that may report veterinary financial data to gain an understanding of your hospital's performance. Bear in mind that regardless of how your hospital data and KPIs compare to industry averages or known benchmarks, what's most important is to evaluate trends in your data. By looking at trends you can assess the growth of the business and compare current performance to prior performance. The best way to evaluate trends is to compare monthly KPIs to the same month from the prior year and to look at changes in monthly numbers during the year.

It is worth noting that when evaluating KPIs, you should consider the impact of the Covid-19 pandemic on your practice. Remember that comparing KPIs such as revenues and new client numbers for 2020 and 2021 to 2019 will likely show substantial increases or decreases depending on how the pandemic affected your community and practice. Some hospitals that experienced an increase in revenues and new clients in 2020 and 2021 may continue to see substantial growth while others might not. Just remember to consider whether any KPIs you look at were pre-pandemic or during the pandemic and continue to closely evaluate trends for your practice.

Total Revenue

Gross revenues include the income from all services and products less any adjustments such as discounts and refunds. Practice revenues correlate with the number of full-time equivalent (FTE) veterinarians in the practice and should therefore increase with the addition of each doctor. Other factors that influence the total practice revenues include the location of the business, median income household income for the area, and years established at the current location. Regardless of the age of the business and demographics of the surrounding area, all practices need to grow to be financially healthy. The percentage growth of a practice should at a minimum increase as much as the annual rate of inflation. This is so the business can maintain the same level of profitability as expenses go up.

Most veterinary practice owners monitor their daily, monthly, and annual gross revenues. This is the easiest KPI to watch because most owners routinely look at the daily and monthly revenue totals for the practice. The amount of revenues relates to whether there is enough cash flow to pay bills, invest in the business and provide a salary for the owner(s). The annual gross revenues indicate the amount of income and revenue growth, but this number doesn't provide significant information about the financial health and profitability of the practice.

When assessing gross revenues, try to figure out what factors correlate to changes in income. You'll be happy if the practice income increases but you want to know why. Revenues may increase due to an influx of new clients or as a result of new service offerings such as grooming and laser therapy. Revenues increase with improved client compliance and when there is an increase in the number of patients seen. But revenue production is also related to fee increases. If revenues only go up because of a price increase implemented the prior month or quarter, there may be no real growth in the practice. This is a problem you want to identify and take action to correct.

You also want to evaluate why revenues go down or remain the same. Has there been a decline in the number of transactions? Is the practice seeing fewer patients? Did the practice lose a doctor or other key team members? Has new client acquisition gone down? How is client compliance for the business? Minor fluctuations in revenues from month to month is not uncommon but if you notice a consistent downward trend in revenues, this is cause for concern. If business revenues are stagnant or declining, there is a clear need to implement marketing action steps to grow the practice.

Of course, KPIs don't always tell the whole story. Be sure to consider external factors that may affect revenues as well. Are you in an area with new housing growth or a well-established neighborhood? Has your community experienced any layoffs for local businesses? Is there road construction nearby that hinders clients' ease of getting to the practice? Is the practice in a shopping center or area that has business closures? What is the state of the economy? The answer to these questions is relevant because you might, for example, view stagnant revenues during a slow economy or recession more favorably than you would during times of economic growth.

Income Categories

Analyzing the amount of income the business receives from the sale of different services and products is important to further assess the financial health of the practice. Looking at the amount of practice income from various service and product categories reveals where the business is making money and can identify areas of opportunity to grow the practice. Specifically, this evaluation helps you better understand which services clients use the most and which ones they might underutilize. To calculate this KPI, divide the revenues for a type of services or product by the total practice revenues to see the amount of income as a percentage of the total hospital revenues.

Managers should evaluate service income categories that are primary profit centers. These include exams/consultations, professional services, vaccinations, surgery, laboratory, diagnostic imaging, dentistry, anesthesia, hospitalization, pharmacy, and flea, tick, and heartworm prevention products. Other income categories that may be relevant for practices include pet food sales, grooming, boarding, and alternative therapies such as acupuncture.

For most small animal practices, service income makes up about two-thirds or more of revenues. This is an important percentage to know because for practices to be financially healthy, service income should be considerably higher than income from product sales. In part, this is because product sales are not as profitable as service sales. Moreover, pet owners have many choices for where to buy products such as pet food, flea, tick, and heartworm preventives as well as over the counter items such as shampoo and supplements. Consumers may shop at online pharmacies and big-box retailers where they may find cheaper prices. As a result, hospital's product sales have trended downward for multiple years. Likewise, pharmacy sales have declined for many hospitals as clients may request prescriptions and then purchase medications at internet pharmacies or another local provider that offers lower cost drugs. To maintain profitability, practices can no longer rely on pharmacy and product sales to be major profit centers.

Managers of specialty and emergency referral hospitals should monitor income categories for the primary services offered to pet owners. These practices don't provide preventive care such as vaccinations, boarding and grooming services, or sell products such as flea, tick, and heartworm preventives. Emergency practices may want to monitor income categories for different levels of hospitalization and critical care. Depending on the specialty services provided, referral hospitals may have expanded income categories for profit centers within their specialty. For example, internal medicine practices may have a separate income category for endoscopy and surgeons may choose to separate orthopedic and soft tissue surgery into two different income categories.

Number of Transactions

The number of transactions refers to the number of invoices for the business. The number of FTE veterinarians affects the total number of transactions. The more doctors, the more transactions. Evaluating the number of transactions is critical because it's an indicator of how the business is doing with new client acquisition, bonding clients, and increasing compliance. For example, when pet owners come back in for recommended blood work and dentistry procedures or refills of medications, the practice generates another invoice. Other factors that increase the number of transactions include whether the practice has grooming, pet daycare, retail sales and technician appointments.

For the practice to grow, transactions need to increase. This is why it's so important to monitor the number of transactions in conjunction with revenues. If revenues increase without an increase in transactions, the most probable cause is a fee increase or possibly an increase in the average transaction charge. Relying only on fee increases to achieve revenue growth isn't sustainable. Likewise, if pet owners feel sticker shock because of the high cost of a single transaction, they may be less likely to schedule future visits. Interestingly, several organizations have data showing it's better for the financial health of the practice to focus on increasing patient visits rather than increasing the amount of each client transaction. Matthew J. Salois, PhD, director of the AVMA Veterinary Economics Division advocates increasing Invoices Per Patient (IPP). AVMA did a study of 400 practices that found a strong correlation between the number of invoices and having a consistently higher overall EBITA. An analysis by the company VetSuccess showed that IPP contributed more to higher revenues than the ATC.[3]

Ideally, the business should attribute transactions to either the hospital or a specific doctor in the PIMS. This distinction becomes relevant when evaluating doctor productivity. Doctor transactions occur whenever veterinarians perform a service or prescribe a medication for a pet. Hospital transactions refers to those invoices with no doctor involvement. This includes the sale of pet food, over-the-counter products, refills on preventive products, grooming, boarding, pet daycare, technician appointments, and refills of medications that don't require doctor involvement.

Average Transaction Charge (ATC)

To calculate the average transaction charge, divide the total hospital revenue by the total number of transactions or invoices. The ATC tends to reflect how the practice team is doing with client recommendations and compliance. The ATC will be higher, for example, when pet owners agree to recommended services such as diagnostics, medications, and preventive products. Bear in mind that if the ATC is low, this may be due to a low fee structure. Note that the ATC is generally lower than the average doctor transaction because it includes all hospital invoices in the calculation even those for small purchases such as sales for one bag of pet food.

Doctor Productivity

Evaluating doctor productivity is important because it directly correlates to the financial success of the business. The veterinarians are responsible for generating most of the revenues and their productivity is a major determinant of the profitability of the business.

Revenue production

Several KPIs assess doctor productivity. One is to compare a doctor's revenue production to industry standards factoring in the number of hours worked. You can find this KPI in reports from the PIMS assuming the business credits invoices to a specific doctor code rather than to the hospital. Clearly, a part-time veterinarian will likely generate less revenues than a full-time doctor. To compare the production for a part-time doctor to industry standards categorize them based on the number of hours worked with 40 hours per week considered as 1.0 FTE. For example, if a doctor works 20 hours a week, she is a 0.5 FTE veterinarian.

Practices should track the amount of revenue doctors generate each month. Changes in doctor production sometimes accounts for why there is a change in the total revenue for the hospital. Practices that pay their doctors a salary without any bonus based on production are sometimes remiss in reviewing doctor production data. Don't make this mistake. Doctors must have adequate revenue production for the hospital to be financially successful. Moreover, it makes sense to ensure that the business compensate veterinarians appropriately based on their revenue production.

Doctor transactions

The second KPI to evaluate is the number of doctor transactions. A low number of doctor transactions indicates a doctor isn't seeing enough clients and patients. Here are questions to consider when faced with this scenario: Is it because business is slow, or because the patient caseload is down for a particular service? Did the veterinarian miss work for some reason? Is the doctor seeing the same number of appointments per day as other doctors? Are they disorganized? Do they have lower compliance rates compared to benchmarks and other doctors in the practice?

Average doctor transaction (ADT)

The third KPI is to look at the average doctor transaction (ADT) for each veterinarian in the practice. This number is determined by diving the total number of invoices generated for a doctor by their revenue production. A higher ADT indicates the veterinarian does an excellent job with case workups and communicating the value of services to pet owners. Veterinarians that perform more surgeries or advanced procedures such as endoscopy and ultrasound may also have a higher ADT.

If you notice a substantial decrease in doctor production or ADT, it's time to investigate the underlying cause for the change. Likewise, if you notice considerable variations in the data for different veterinarians in the practice, see if you can find out why one doctor is able to produce more than his or her colleague.

Team Productivity

By measuring team productivity, managers can determine the level of efficiency for the hospital and evaluate the efficiency for different days and team members. One way to evaluate team productivity is to look at the number of hours worked compared to the number of hospital transactions. To calculate this KPI divide both the average number of staff hours and the average number of DVM hours per period by the total number of transactions for the same period. Then add the number of staff hours per transaction to the number of DVM hours per transaction to determine the average total hours per transaction.

The target goals are to have 1.0-1.5 staff hours per transaction and 0.3-0.5 DVM hours per transaction.[4] There are few published benchmarks for the hours per transaction but here are performance ratings that have been reported for the average total number of hours per transaction:

- 1.3 hours per transaction is superior performance.
- 1. 5 to 1.75 hours per transaction is good performance
- 1.75 to 2.0 hours per transaction is average
- 2.0 to 2.25 hours per transaction is below average

Bear in mind that you want the support staff hours per transaction to be higher than the doctor hours. To increase team productivity, first make sure the practice is fully leveraging the use of support staff before hiring another doctor. If there are variations in efficiency for different days of the week or when different team members are working, further exploration is warranted. Questions to consider include:

- Why are some team members more efficient?
- Which doctors and staff members see more clients and patients?
- Do all employees follow the same protocols?
- Can scheduling be modified to improve efficiency for all days of the week?
- Are there any problems with team conflict or employee engagement during specific shifts during the workweek?
- Is there the same amount of support staff working on all days of the week?
- Are doctors doing tasks or procedures that could be done by support staff?

The number of patients seen per doctor per hour is another way to measure practice efficiency. This metric became more obvious in 2021 when AVMA reported that veterinarians saw fewer patients per hour and declines of almost 25% in practice productivity in 2020 compared to 2019.[5] The decline was no doubt due to the many challenges related to the COVID-19 pandemic such as staff shortages, changes in safety protocols and the need to transition to curbside care to deliver services. Looking at trends in the number of patients seen per doctor and comparing data for different doctors and days of the week is an important evaluation for practices that need to improve efficiency.

Another evaluation of team productivity is the staff/DVM ratio. To measure this ratio, divide the number of full time equivalent (FTE) non-DVM staff by the number of FTE equivalent DVMs. You can also calculate the KPI by dividing the total support staff hours by the total number of DVM appointment/surgery hours in a specific time period. Decisions about the amount of team members to schedule each day is one of the greatest challenges for managers. Doctors and non-DVM staff alike both want as many co-workers as possible because it can make everyone's job easier. From a business standpoint, managers must control staff expenses to maintain profitability. But with too few staff, doctors can't be efficient and may not be able to meet the demands of clients or provide all the care patients need.

Looking at the staff to doctor ratio in combination with other KPIs can help you make assessments about team productivity. A low staff to doctor ratio may be a primary reason for low doctor productivity, a high number of hours per transaction and a decline in the number of patients seen by doctors. On the other hand, if you have an average or above average staff/DVM ratio (such as 4.5:1 or greater) and still have low team productivity then you want to look for other solutions to increase productivity besides adding more team members.

New Clients and Patients

A new client is defined as one that purchases a product or service from the practice for the first time. Practices should track the number of new clients monthly. The benchmark for the number of new clients per month is based on the number of FTE doctors in the practice. Presumably, the more doctors, the greater the number of new clients.

Historically multiple veterinary sources have reported the ideal number of new clients per month per FTE doctor to be 25-30. However, there has been a decline in the average number of new clients per month in recent years for many hospitals. AAHA reported an average of 28 new clients per month per FTE doctor in 2007 and an average of 21 new clients per month FTE doctor in 2009 and 2011. 2017 data from AAHA shows an average of 22 new clients per month.[6] In 2019, the Well Managed Practices Benchmarks® study[7] reported the number of new clients per doctor at 18 per month but previously reported the number at 22 per month in 2008 and 20 per month in 2009. Data from the monthly Insider's Insights VHMA report showed a decline in the growth of new clients for practices for multiple years.[8]

It is noteworthy that starting in 2020 and continuing into the first quarter of 2021, both VHMA and VetSuccess reports revealed a significant increase in the number of new clients each month. This trend started during the COVID-19 pandemic. Given the high unemployment rates and economic hardship for many people, this was initially a surprise for the profession. However, it became apparent that the rise in new client numbers for practices were likely a result of increased pet adoptions, clients not being able to get in to see their regular veterinarian due to closures or understaffing, an enhanced awareness of pets' needs by pet owners staying at home, more discretionary income spent on veterinary care instead of other costs such as dining out and travel. When evaluating new client numbers, managers should look at trends for several years factoring in that the increases seen in 2020-2021 may or may not persist in future years.

Practices need to attract new clients each month to maintain and enhance the financial success of the business. This is because of the inevitable attrition of clients that occurs related to people moving, the death of pets, and clients deciding to switch to a different hospital. The acquisition of new clients each year needs to exceed the number of clients who are lost for the business to grow.

Practice managers should endeavor to evaluate factors contributing to the number of new clients each month and assess this KPI in conjunction with other revenue data. Just because the business doesn't meet or exceed the benchmark for new client numbers doesn't mean the practice isn't doing well. For example, a practice located in a well-established area with no new growth may see fewer new clients than a practice in an area that has new housing developments. On the other hand, a practice located near a military base or in an area of retirement communities may have high new client numbers. By itself, this doesn't mean the practice is doing well because not all these new clients will stay with the practice long-term.

When evaluating new client numbers, managers should look at monthly trends for new clients and compare the number of new clients per month to the same month the prior year. A downward trend in new client acquisition is cause for concern. However, a seasonal decrease that is consistent each year may not be noteworthy. Additionally, the source of referrals needs to be tracked for all new clients which helps with marketing planning. Team members should enter this information in the practice management software when new clients are checked in.

Relevant factors that can contribute to a low number of new clients per month include ineffective external marketing efforts, competition, insufficient word of mouth referrals, failure to convert potential client calls and lack of community presence. Chapter 10 on Marketing and Client Communications presents action steps to address these challenges.

A new patient is one that is seen for the first time by the hospital. Both existing clients and new clients present new patients. Just as with new clients, the hospital growth depends on new patients. One way to grow the number of new patients is to ensure that all pets in a household are receiving appropriate care. We know feline visits to veterinarians are lower than canine visits. By asking "What other pets live with you?" or "What furry friends does Hannah have at home?" you may discover new patients to provide care for.

Client Retention and Client Visitation

The measure for client retention, sometimes referred to as the bonding rate, is calculated by dividing the number of active clients by the number of new clients. This KPI shows how bonded pet owners are to the practice, so you want to look at it along with the number of new clients. If the practice has a high number of new clients but low client retention, this may indicate the need for a better client experience.

The client visitation rate is a measure of how many times an active client visits the hospital each year. It's an indicator of how well the practice is doing with client retention and compliance. To calculate this KPI, divide the number of annual transactions by the number of active clients. The target goal is to have a client visitation rate of 2.0-3.0 visits per year.

Active Clients and Patients

Active clients are defined as those clients that have purchased a service or product within the past year. Some organizations define this KPI using an 18-month period. Likewise, the number of active patients refers to patients that have been seen at least once in the last 12-18 months. The number of active clients and patients directly correlates with how well the business is doing in getting clients in the hospital, so their pets receive appropriate care.

The number of active clients may decline when clients move out of the area, switch hospitals or are unhappy with your services. The number of active clients and patients is also a reflection of the effectiveness of the business's reminder system and client compliance rates.

Client Compliance

Practices can derive compliance statistics by calculating the percentage of utilization for a service or product based on the number of pets who need the service or product. Compliance rates are evaluated to determine how well pet owners comply with medical recommendations. Calculating compliance requires extracting data from the PIMS and can be tedious. Multiple companies can assist practices by extracting this data and providing reports to the management team. Whether you calculate compliance rates on your own or with the assistance of an outside party, establish goals along with action steps to improve.

You can view pet owner compliance from two perspectives. One view is that compliance rates show how well pet owners adhere to recommendations from the veterinary team. Do they come in for annual exams and recommended vaccinations? Do they keep their dogs on year-round heartworm prevention as recommended by the American Heartworm Society?[9] Do they say yes to recommendations for preventive care laboratory testing? Do they come in for recommended dental care procedures?

The other way to view compliance is from the perspective of how well the team is doing at communicating the value of services and products. Do pet owners appreciate the need and the value of recommendations? We know from surveys and studies that pet owner compliance with recommendations is a challenge for practices. In Chapter 10 on Marketing and Client Communications you will find action steps to improve compliance.

Setting Goals to Improve

Evaluating data and KPIs isn't enough to achieve financial success. The key to practice growth and enhancing profitability is setting goals to improve. When tracking metrics, consider these questions:

- How is the practice doing compared to other similar businesses?
- How is the practice doing compared to previous months?
- What action steps can be implemented to improve the financial health of the business?

The last question above is critical. The role of practice owners and managers is to use KPIs as a foundation to set hospital goals and implement specific tactics to achieve these goals. If the business is underperforming, set goals to improve in those areas that you identify as priorities or that show the greatest opportunity for improving profitability. Even if the business has favorable KPIs compared to industry averages, the question should be "Do you want to just be average?" Every practice can and should set target goals to improve the financial position of the business.

A major goal for most practice owners is to increase revenues. Assuming cost control measures, this could be the best way to increase profitability. There are only so many ways to increase revenues. To easily see your options to grow revenues, consult Figure 9.1 to consider which opportunities might be best for the business. You can read more about the actions to grow revenues shown in the chart in the next chapter on marketing. Not every tactic will work well for every business. For example, it may be difficult to add a new doctor if the practice can't recruit one. And adding a new doctor doesn't automatically mean the number of transactions will increase. Managers would need to implement plans aimed at filling the appointment schedule for the new veterinarian. Likewise, team training may or may not increase compliance depending on the quality of the training and the team's ability to improve client communications.

Figure 9.1: How to Grow Practice Revenue

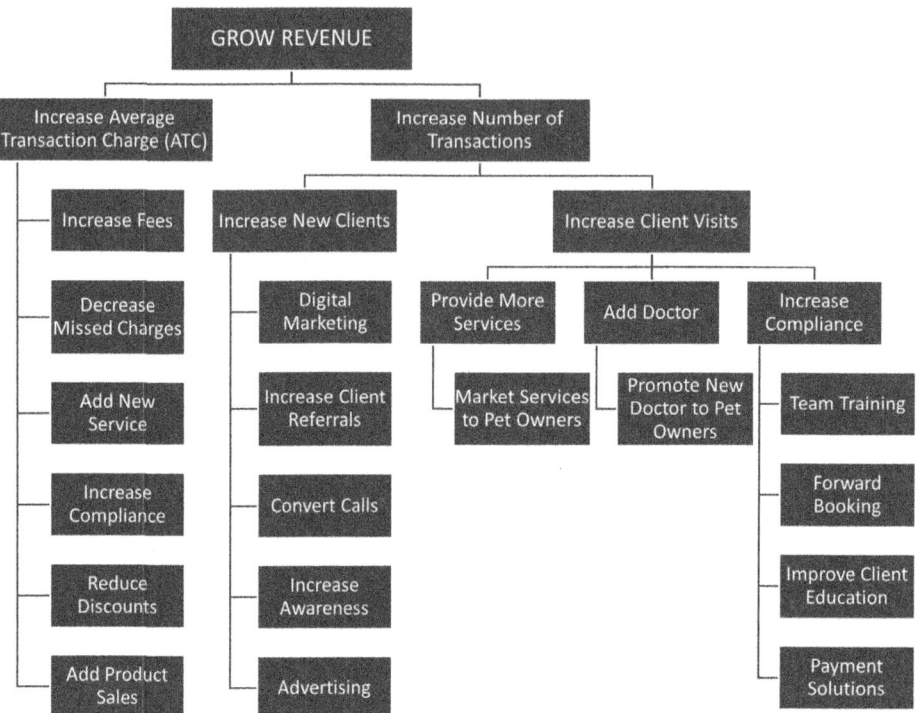

UNDERSTANDING PROFIT & LOSS STATEMENTS

While some managers evaluate monthly Profit & Loss (P&L) statements, others may never look at these reports. Regardless of your level of involvement, all managers benefit from understanding the basics of reading a P&L statement. Typically, managers generate a P&L statement at the end of each month and at the end of the year, but you can view a profit and loss report for any time period. If the practice owner, practice manager or the hospital's bookkeeper is entering the hospital data into an accounting software program such as Quickbooks, the P&L is easily accessible at any time. However, if the practice outsources this accounting job to the business's accountant, then the P&L is often not available until 4-6 weeks past the end of the month.

The P&L statement shows the business income, expenses, and net income. These statements group expenses into major categories for both fixed and variable expenses. Fixed expenses are those incurred regardless of the number of patients seen. These are overhead expenses that are essentially "the cost of doing business." Fixed expenses are relatively consistent from month to month and don't fluctuate much regardless of the revenue of the practice. Fixed expenses include costs such as rent or loan payments, utilities, phone, IT support, worker's compensation premiums, all insurance payments, property taxes, continuing education, uniforms, professional services fees, marketing fees and management salaries. Variable expenses are those that change in relation to the number of patients seen. Variable expenses include costs such as drugs, preventives, medical supplies, laboratory supplies and fees, cremations, merchant/credit card fees, food and retail products, sales tax, and rabies tags.

The largest expenses for a practice are doctor and staff wages, cost of goods sold and facilities expenses. Cost of goods sold (COGS) includes the expense for all drugs, medical supplies, lab and imaging costs, cremations, and pet food. The facilities expense includes rent, hospital maintenance and repairs, utilities, property tax, and business insurance.

A review of the P&L statement is more meaningful if the report includes a column that shows the expenses as a percentage of the total income. This helps show the major expenses for the business and allows for comparison to industry benchmarks that have been established for most expense categories. You can also include a column that shows values for the prior year which then helps show whether expenses have gone up, down or stayed the same.

Part of the value of evaluating the practice's P&L statements is being able to compare whether the hospital's expenses are consistent with industry averages and benchmarks reported for profitable practices. However, if you or your accountant aren't using accounting classification codes for income and expenses according to veterinary industry standards, it's difficult to measure your practice's performance against known benchmarks. Ideally, standardized veterinary accounting codes should be used because they allow practice owners to better organize their financials and analyze data to improve the organization. To be able to make accurate comparisons, you and your accountant can work together to use the AAHA/VMG Chart of Accounts. You can download these documents from AAHA's website. It is the standard for classifying and aggregating revenue, expense, and balance sheet accounts in small-animal veterinary practice.[10] Multiple veterinary organizations and industry partners recommend and endorse this chart of accounts including AVMA, VHMA, and VetPartners, which is a national group of veterinary consultants and advisors.

Expense Control

One of the most important job roles of a manager is to control costs. Even if you don't review the monthly P&L statements, ask the practice owner to share with you how the business is doing with expense control. If expenses go up or exceed established industry benchmarks, try to determine the underlying cause so you can implement action steps to lower the expense. The three largest expense categories are payroll, cost of goods sold, and facility expenses. As such, these expenses can have a significant impact on profitability for the business.

Facility expenses

Facility costs include the business's rent or mortgage payment, property taxes, business insurance, hospital repairs and maintenance, and utilities. If the rent payment is to a third party that doesn't own the practice, it may be possible to renegotiate the lease when it comes due. Practice leaders can check each year to make sure they're getting the best rates for business insurance. Since the facility expenses are mostly fixed costs, the best way to decrease this expense is to grow the practice by increasing income which will bring down the facility expense as a percentage of total income.

Let's look at why expenses may be too high for payroll and COGS and action steps you could take to lower these expenses.

Cost of goods sold (COGS)

If the COGS is high, the primary cause is usually poor inventory management. Think of all your drugs, medical supplies, flea/tick/heartworm preventives and pet food as "cash on the shelves." You wouldn't leave cash laying around! You don't want more inventory in the building than you need. The goal is to have sufficient inventory to meet the needs of patients without overstocking. You also don't want to run out of inventory. Ideally, the inventory turnover should occur 8-12 times per year. This means products would only sit on the shelf 30-45 days. Since most practices can order and receive inventory within a few days, you may only need to stock enough inventory to last a week or two.

Utilizing your practice management software's inventory component can help track quantities on hand, usage, purchase orders as well as control markups and cost increases from suppliers. Unfortunately, many practices underutilize this functionality and inventory counts are inaccurate. If this is true for your practice, it's worth spending time to learn about the software and how you can take advantage of it to improve efficiency and improve inventory control.

Regardless of whether you fully utilize your practice management software for inventory management or do manual counts to put together a purchase order, you must establish a desired quantity on hand and re-order points for all inventory items. This can be a tedious job, but it's well worth the time spent to achieve what will likely be substantial cost savings.

Other causes of high COGS include carrying too many duplicate products, mark-ups that are too low, taking advantage of too many promotions resulting in overstocking and inventory shrinkage. Inventory shrinkage refers to the loss of inventory that may occur due to damage, miscounting or theft.

Staff and doctor payroll

There are many factors that influence the cost of payroll. Therefore, managers should evaluate all the reasons why this expense may be high. First, look at staff compensation. Is everyone paid according to wages that are consistent for the veterinary industry and your region? Are highly compensated employees providing value to the hospital? For example, a credentialled veterinary technician with experience may be highly compensated. Does this employee help generate revenue because of the procedures they're able to perform and services they provide to patients? Unfortunately, sometimes hospitals have long-term employees who are highly compensated because they receive raises every year, but they aren't productive. When this happens, payroll costs go up without a corresponding benefit to the business. Excessive overtime can be a cause of high staff payroll costs especially if the most highly compensated team members are the ones getting overtime. (See Table 9.1 to assess possible causes of high support staff payroll.)

Next evaluate doctor compensation. Practices pay full-time doctors a salary or some type of production-based pay. Doctors on production usually receive compensation equal to somewhere between 16 and 25 percent of their revenue production. Regardless of the compensation model used to pay doctors, industry experts and consultants agree the total amount paid for compensation and benefits shouldn't exceed 25 percent of what they produce in revenue in order for the practice to be profitable.[11]

Other causes of high payroll expenses include issues related to operations and human resource management such as overstaffing, operational inefficiency, a lack of team productivity and having a high staff to doctor ratio. Remember that a high staff to doctor ratio isn't necessarily a cause of high payroll if the team is highly productive and can see more patients and clients.

Even though facility expenses, payroll and COGS are the primary expenses to monitor, this doesn't mean managers should ignore the rest of the expenses. Even small changes to other expenses can add up to significant cost savings. An example is credit card fees. If credit card fees are higher than 1.8-2%, it may be worth investigating other processing companies to see if you can lower this expense and save thousands of dollars.

Table 9.1: Assessing Causes of High Support Staff Payroll

Possible Causes	Questions to Consider
Overtime	• Which employees have overtime: is it a few or across the board? • Are employees clocking in and out as expected? • Does the business need to recruit additional employees?
Overstaffing	• Evaluate work schedules: are employees scheduled according to the business needs? • Are there seasonal changes for staffing needs?
High staff to doctor ratio	• Does the ratio exceed industry averages? • Are employees always busy? • Are team members productive?
Highly compensated employees	• Are team members helping produce revenues? • Are raises given without merit?
Lack of team productivity	• Does the practice have problems with efficiency? • Are some employees more productive than others?
Decrease in revenues	• How much have revenues declined and for how long? • Is the decrease due to a decline in transactions? • Has the business raised fees each year and as costs increase?

PRICING STRATEGIES

A pricing strategy refers to the method used to determine the best price for services and products that maximizes revenues and profit for the company while ensuring the business maintains a competitive position in the marketplace. The pricing strategy for a veterinary practice needs to take into consideration multiple internal and external factors about the business. These may include the practice location, hospital appearance, quality of care, expertise of the team, service mix, local economy, consumer demand, and level of competition. Moreover, the pricing strategy needs to consider what pet owners can realistically pay for veterinary care and what they are willing to pay which correlates with their perceived value of services and products. Bear in mind practices may use multiple pricing strategies depending on the type of service or product.

Developing and implementing an effective pricing strategy helps grow the business, enhance profitability, and ensure client satisfaction. A pricing strategy isn't just about how and when to increase fees. Fee increases can help grow revenues and make sure the business's income keeps pace with rising costs. This in turn can positively affect profitability. However, raising fees as the only means to increase revenues is not a sustainable business strategy to enhance growth and profitability.

One of the essential elements of your pricing strategy is to make sure fees are consistent with the business model for the practice. Does the practice compete primarily based on price? Hospitals that are lower-cost providers strive to attract and retain clients by promoting affordable or low fees compared to other practices. The pricing strategy for these businesses is to have fees that are lower than other hospitals in the area. At the other end of the spectrum, specialty and emergency referral hospitals offer advanced diagnostics, medical treatments, and surgery. Their pricing strategy is based on the value of the services as well as the cost to provide the care which is why these hospitals have higher fees than general practices.

Another relevant aspect of a pricing strategy is to decide if the business wants to be a price leader, price follower, have lower fees, or always stay in the middle of the pack with fees. None of these strategies is right or wrong. But take care to make a conscious decision about the pricing strategy and why it makes sense for the business. For example, if the practice is in an area with a diverse client base that includes pet owners from different economic neighborhoods, it may not make sense to adopt a price leader pricing strategy.

Market-Based Pricing

Let's look at some different pricing strategies starting with market-based pricing. With this strategy, practices endeavor to set fees that are consistent with what their colleagues or other area practices charge for the same service or product. This strategy has its limitations since there are only a few ways to know what other practices charge. You must be cautious when talking to area managers to avoid charges of "price-fixing." Alternatively, you can look at published data such as The Veterinary Fee Reference book from AAHA which includes information about hundreds of common fees.[12] When comparing your fees to those charged by other hospitals, be mindful of making an apples-to-apples comparison which isn't always easy. Your practice might be different than the other practices in many ways and you may charge for your services differently.

Cost-Based Pricing

Another pricing strategy is the cost-based pricing strategy. With cost-based pricing, businesses determine what the costs are to provide a service and what fee to charge so the business makes a profit. It's relatively easy to do cost-based pricing for products because the cost to purchase the product from a vendor is known. The staff costs related to inventory management are relatively easy to calculate and the last step is to just decide on the desired markup to make a profit. However, using a cost-based pricing strategy for services is more difficult. You need to calculate the cost of all medical supplies, overhead costs and equipment costs related to the service, and the employee compensation costs including payroll taxes and benefits of the doctors and staff based on their time to provide the service. Even though this pricing strategy is time consuming and involves more detailed analysis, it's wise to always try to evaluate the cost of providing services. Otherwise, profitability for the business may suffer.

Value-Based Pricing

The next pricing strategy frequently advocated in veterinary medicine is the values-based pricing strategy. Value-based pricing is based on determining what clients are willing to pay for a service or product based on the value it provides. This strategy doesn't ignore the cost of providing the service nor does it mean fees are set at the highest price a client might pay. As an example, consider the fee for an otic cytology. The cost to provide this service is minimal. The only medical supplies are a cotton swab, microscope slide, small amount of stain and immersion oil. The only equipment used is the microscope. The time for a team member to collect the sample, stain the slide and read the cytology is likely no more than 10 minutes. Let's say you find the cost of supplies and labor to provide the service is $4.50. Even with a 300% markup, the fee would only be $13.50 which is considerably lower than what most practices charge for this service. Charging a higher fee makes sense based on the expertise needed to evaluate the cytology and the value of the service, which is to diagnose the type and severity of infections. However, if the fee is too high, client compliance goes down.

The values-based strategy can be the ideal strategy, but it's more difficult to implement because you have to think about what the client thinks the service or product is worth, not just what practice leaders think it's worth. The hospital team may appreciate the time, expertise, and equipment that it takes to provide a service whereas the client may not. Helping clients understand the cost of care is one of the reasons why everyone in the practice needs to be able to clearly communicate the value of your services and products to pet owners. Remember, the client experience is also a major contributing factor to perceived value for pet owners. Clients value the medical care but also value how they're treated, the hospital environment and whether it's convenient to do business with the practice. Consumers are willing to pay higher fees when they have an exceptional client experience.

Given the complexity of determining pricing for veterinary services, practice leaders may want to use a combination of strategies. Market-based pricing, for example, makes sense for commonly utilized services such as preventive care and dentistry. Values-based pricing may be used for many of the services provided to sick patients. When pricing surgeries, a cost-based strategy may be the best, so the business doesn't lose money when performing major procedures. What's most important is for practice leaders to thoughtfully evaluate what strategies make the most sense for their business.

Setting Fees

Regardless of what pricing strategy the practice adopts, fee increases help to maintain and enhance profitability. This means most practices need to routinely increase fees 2-4% just to cover rising costs and keep up with inflation. Evaluate fees at a minimum once or twice a year to see if adjustments should be made. Most practices implement fee increases annually or twice a year. When hospitals raise fees twice a year, often this is because practice leaders decided to split the fee increase into two time periods. For example, instead of increasing fees by 5% in January, the business increases fees 2.5% in January and again in June. The idea behind this approach is that clients are less likely to notice a smaller fee increase. The disadvantage is the loss of revenue because of waiting six months for the second fee increase. When implementing fee increases, most companion animal practices strive to make sure their fees for "shopped" services and products are competitive with area hospitals. This includes all the commonly quoted fees pet owners inquire about such as exams, vaccinations, heartworm and fecal tests, sterilization surgeries and flea/tick/heartworm preventives.

Part of having an effective pricing strategy and process for setting fees is for managers to stay organized. This means keeping track of any adjustments to fees, so you have an historical record of your actions. You can use a spreadsheet to show the date of fee increases, the percentage increase or dollar amount change for fees and which fees were adjusted. Keeping track of fee adjustments helps practice leaders make informed decisions about when and how much to raise fees. Moreover, knowing when the practice increased fees may be relevant when evaluating KPIs such as the number of transactions, new client numbers and compliance rates. And don't forget to inform the team when increasing fees so they're prepared to respond if clients notice. (See textbox "Explaining Fee Increases to Clients.")

A final note about fees is for managers to make sure they have protocols in place to avoid missed charges. Failing to capture all fees on the client's invoice can result in a substantial decrease in revenues for the practice. The first step is to periodically conduct an audit by comparing medical charts against invoices to identify if there are any missed charges. To ensure the accuracy of invoices, it's best if the practice has protocols in place such as using travel sheets to record charges as services are performed and having two employees check invoices for accuracy before clients pay.

UNDERSTANDING PRACTICE PROFITABILITY

Practice profitability is unquestionably one of the most important performance indicators for your business, but it is not an easy calculation. This is not the amount shown as net income on a P&L or tax return. The true profitability is determined by making some adjustments for non-operating and/or non-recurring expenses, fair market rent and fair market salary for the owner. Some people refer to profitability as EBITDA (earnings before interest, taxes, depreciation, amortization).

Practice profitability is critical because it directly correlates with the value of the practice. Companies that value veterinary practices consider a practice to be financially healthy if it's 14-18% profitable. Unfortunately, many practices may only be 10-12% profitable and some fall into the category of what the organization VetPartners termed a "no-low" practice meaning the business has no or low profits.[13] When veterinary practice owners are ready to sell their business, it can be disconcerting if not devastating to discover it isn't worth the value they assumed they would get for the business.

> **EXPLAINING FEE INCREASES TO CLIENTS**
>
> Clients often don't notice fee increases. But when they do, team members should be ready to respond to their questions or comments with positive, consistent messages.
>
> Managers should always alert team members when there is going to be a fee increase and explain the reasons for the change in prices. Most employees as well as clients understand fee increases are necessary to maintain the practice's financial health and to keep pace with increasing costs of drugs, supplies, and overhead. But just telling clients, "Our costs have gone up, so we increased prices" won't necessarily be well received. Instead, teams should focus on patient advocacy and the value of services. A more positive message is to say phrases such as, "We increased some of our fees so we can continue to provide high-quality medical care for pets and outstanding service to our clients. We don't like to raise fees, but we're committed to excellence."
>
> Most importantly, teams should reinforce the value of services with statements such as, "I know Ginger's medical care is expensive at times and we appreciate that you take such good care of her. The blood work we're doing today will help us assess her internal organ function and make sure she's healthy before we start her on long-term medications for her arthritis."
>
> Clients are more likely to accept and understand fee increases when team members convey messages that focus on patient advocacy and the human-pet bond.

Practice owners shouldn't be lulled into a false sense of security just because they can pay their bills and take home a salary. Instead, they should consistently monitor the practice profitability and take steps to increase profitability if evaluations determine the business isn't financially healthy. Working with trusted advisors such as accountants, financial planners, practice valuators and consultants on a regular basis is especially beneficial if owners intend to sell the business within 5 years. Savvy business owners understand and live by the motto "it's never too early to plan your exit strategy."

SUMMARY

After reading this chapter, you should have a clear understanding of the importance of financial management and know which key performance indicators to monitor on a regular basis. As noted previously, even if you aren't responsible for evaluating hospital data it's still important to know how the business is performing compared to industry benchmarks. Even more importantly, you should be aware of trends in KPIs as they indicate how the practice is doing in terms of growth and profitability. Regardless of the current financial position of the business, practice leaders should consistently strive to maximize growth potential, enhance profitability, and stay competitive in the marketplace. Which leads to the next chapter on marketing. You can use the information you've gleaned about financial management to help formulate the right marketing goals for your practice.

CHAPTER 10

Marketing and Client Communications

When asked to define marketing, veterinary professionals give a variety of answers. Some mention advertising or say marketing is getting the word out about the practice. Others reference having a digital presence and website. Many people equate marketing to the importance of delivering excellent client service, attracting clients, communicating the value of services, or building client loyalty. These are all correct answers and speak to the fact that marketing is a broad term that encompasses a large scope of business activities.

The American Marketing Association approved this definition of marketing in 2017: "Marketing is the activity, set of institutions, and processes for creating, communicating, delivering, and exchanging offerings that have value for customers, clients, partners, and society at large."[1] Consider this simplified version of the definition for veterinary medicine: "Marketing is the activities and processes used by veterinary practices to create, communicate, and deliver services and products that have value for clients and the community."

The key word when thinking about marketing is "value" because people don't like to pay for a service or product unless it has value to them. Moreover, *how much* a consumer is willing to spend depends on how much value they place on the service or product. The value of a hamburger from a fast-food drive-through restaurant is convenience and low cost whereas the value of dining at an upscale steakhouse is the quality of the food, the ambience, and the service. People are willing to pay much more for a night out if they have an exceptional dining experience.

How businesses create and deliver value depends on whether the company offers primarily services or only sells products. The difference is largely because products are tangible, and services are intangible. If someone buys a high quality, 65 inch, flat-screen TV, they can appreciate the large screen and amazing color every night. The features of the TV are what is important; this includes the size, high-definition picture, and the ability to connect to an online streaming video service. On the other hand, if a pet owner spends the same amount of money on dentistry care, they don't have a tangible product to take home and evaluate. They can't take home the anesthesia, injectable medications, dental radiographs, or dental cleaning. Instead, pet owners appreciate the relationships and experiences associated with their purchase. Pet owners value interacting with a trusted healthcare team and knowing their beloved companion is pain-free and healthier.

The fundamental question to always ask when deciding how to market your veterinary practice is "What do pet owners value?" People love their pets so marketing activities should focus on client communications and client education aimed at promoting the human-animal bond and helping more pets get care. Remember, when people buy services, value is tied to their feelings and the memory of the service experience. Going back to the fine dining experience--why would someone pay so much for food they only enjoyed once? It's because of the positive feelings and shared memories that can last a long time. The same is true for veterinary service expenditures. Clients pay for healthcare for their beloved companions because they want to be great pet parents and keep their pets with them as long as possible. Of course, pet owners must understand the value of services (and products) sold by veterinary hospitals before they visit the practice and before they say "yes" to our services.

MARKETING STRATEGY

Marketing strategy can be defined as your business's comprehensive plan to promote and sell services and products to pet owners. More specifically, marketing strategy is about identifying and focusing on the best opportunities to grow your business and stay competitive. To execute the best marketing plan, take a step back and think about the big picture. Too often, practice leaders engage in multiple marketing activities and launch initiatives without first developing an organized, strategic plan. If you've ever thought "I need to do some marketing for the practice" then you might want to change that thought to "What are the best ways to market our practice?" Well-thought-out marketing plans have a greater chance of success. Here are good questions for the leadership team to discuss:

- What did the strategic planning process reveal? (See "Strategic Planning" in Chapter 2.)
- How can we differentiate our hospital?
- Do pet owners in the community know our values and what we stand for?
- What's working well and what's not working well for our clients?

- Who are our target markets?
- What do we need to do to provide more value to pet owners?
- How can we help pet owners better understand the value of our services and products?

Evaluate KPIs

You can find the best opportunities to grow the business by evaluating KPIs. In chapter 9, you learned the key to practice growth and enhancing profitability is to evaluate KPIs and then set goals to improve the financial success of the business. (See Figure 9.2: How to Grow Revenue.) This analysis helps to distinguish which marketing goals make the most sense for your practice. The number of new clients, number of transactions, ADT, percentages for service utilization, and compliance rates are all good indicators of how the business is doing with marketing efforts. Having said this, even after evaluating KPIs, you may still feel like marketing is a daunting challenge. After all, isn't there always an opportunity to improve all KPIs? What do you do if the practice is underperforming in multiple areas? The key to your success is to decide on marketing plan priorities.

Establishing priorities may be based on multiple factors. One is the practice's available resources which includes money, time, and labor. If cash flow is tight, you may need to implement less costly marketing initiatives. Another consideration is to look at which marketing efforts benefit the greatest number of patients. For example, focusing on marketing initiatives to increase utilization for dentistry services makes sense because so many pets in the practice need oral care. Other factors to assess when determining priorities include the expertise of the team, which marketing plans deliver what clients value most, and which initiatives will result in the greatest growth for the business.

Internal And External Marketing

Marketing strategies should include the right balance of internal and external marketing. External marketing is all activities aimed at attracting new clients. These initiatives are critical since veterinary practices need to acquire new clients due to the inevitable client attrition that occurs when people move or switch hospitals. Internal marketing focuses on leveraging the talent of the team to increase service and product utilization from the practice's existing client base. These strategies include enhancing client service, engagement, loyalty, and compliance as well as improving team training.

Internal marketing is often considered to be of greater importance because you already have an established relationship with your existing clients. Theoretically, it should be easier to market services and products to existing clients than to pet owners who don't know about the practice. Moreover, access to current clients makes it's easier to leverage multiple client communication methods to increase client engagement, loyalty, and compliance.

Deciding how much time and money to spend on internal vs. external marketing depends on the age of the business, its location, the business model, growth phase of the practice, and an evaluation of the hospital's KPIs. However, it's never a good idea to become complacent about external marketing since practices need a consistent number of new clients each month to maintain long-term success and profitability.

Focus on Target Markets

Targeting specific markets is part of having a comprehensive marketing strategy. Target markets are groups of pet owners the practice wishes to attract and/or serve. For most practices, the largest target market is all pet owners in a reasonable geographic area surrounding the practice. Marketing is more effective when target markets are further divided by market segmentation which refers to dividing markets into smaller groups based on specific criteria. Pet owners may be identified based on characteristics such as zip code, age, gender, species of pet owned, and desired services. You might, for example, target millennial pet owners, people who own cats, clients with senior pets, or pet owners in a specific community. Marketing segmentation increases the effectiveness of marketing initiatives because it's more personalized and easier to measure results when targeting a smaller group of people. Most veterinary marketing companies that provide reminder solutions offer targeted marketing via emails or push notifications (messages that pops up on a mobile device).

ESTABLISHING MARKETING GOALS

After deciding on the marketing strategy, the next step is to set clearly defined marketing goals. An effective process to follow is that of setting SMART goals. George T. Doran is generally credited with first writing about smart goals in his paper, "There's a S.M.A.R.T. way to write management's goals and objectives" published in the Management Review in 1981. The acronym is used to help ensure goals are clear and actionable. Each goal should be:

- **S**pecific (simple, sensible, significant)
- **M**easurable (meaningful, motivating)

- **A**chievable (agreed, attainable)
- **R**elevant (reasonable, realistic, and resourced, results-based)
- **T**ime bound (time-based, time limited, time/cost limited, timely, time-sensitive)[2]

Problems can arise with marketing if goals are too broad and vague. Consider a marketing goal of increasing dentistry revenues or dental compliance. While this is an excellent goal, how will you know if you achieve results? Using the SMART goal process, here's how you could define the goal:

- Specific: Increase the number of scheduled dentistry procedures for each month.
- Measurable: Schedule 3 more dentistry procedures per week or increase dental revenues by 20% each month. (Notice there is a number attached to the goal.)
- Achievable: The team has discussed and agreed upon the goal.
- Relevant: The goal is a stretch but still reasonable.
- Time bound: The goal is monthly, and results will be posted for the team to track their progress.

As stated earlier, ideally marketing goals should align with information gleaned from the practice's KPIs. Explaining KPIs to the team helps them understand the rationale for the goal and know the starting point for initiatives. Again, looking at dentistry, everyone can agree that if only 4% of the hospital's service income comes from dentistry, then not nearly enough pets are receiving appropriate dental care.

A common pitfall occurs when leadership teams are overly ambitious and set an unrealistic number of goals. It's far better to focus on a few goals at a time. Practices that focus on a reasonable number of goals each quarter are more likely to be successful attaining goals than practices that try to do too much. Remember team members may feel overwhelmed and frustrated if they're asked to achieve too many goals or focus on too many actions steps at a time.

IMPLEMENTING MARKETING PLANS

Once marketing goals are defined, it's time to implement the marketing plan. Ready, set, go! But wait a minute. If it's that easy, why do some practices struggle with their marketing initiatives? In many instances, it's because the marketing objectives don't have detailed tactics. Without tactics, marketing goals quickly become more of a wish or desire as opposed to an attainable goal.

Developing Tactics

Tactics are the detailed action steps taken to achieve marketing goals. Tactics should clearly define *how* to implement the tactic, *who* will act, and *when* actions will take place. For the goal of increasing the number of dental procedures per week, one tactic might be to better communicate the value of dental care to clients. The "how" could be for team members to convey one or more benefit statements about dentistry when making recommendations. The "who" applies to all team members who make recommendations and the "when" includes communicating value when presenting dental care treatment plans.

Just as with goals, it's best to focus on implementing a few tactics at one time. Let's say, for example, the business has a goal to increase the number of new clients each month. It isn't reasonable to try to launch a client referral program, plan a community event to promote awareness, and implement a phone skills training program all in the same month. Likewise, asking employees to improve client compliance by using five new exam room communication skills during every appointment is asking for trouble. A more realistic approach is to have the team focus on one or two communications at a time.

Measuring Success

Don't forget to measure the success of your marketing initiatives. No one wants to spend money or energy on marketing efforts that don't yield results for the business. To measure the success of marketing goals, you can evaluate changes in specific KPIs and compliance rates as well as client satisfaction. Be sure to calculate the return on investment for all major marketing expenditures. To do this, total the amount of money spent on marketing as well as time involved and make certain that the amount of revenue generated or the number of new clients gained was positive. Remember it may take multiple months to see the results of marketing tactics. A review of quarterly and year-end data can help you decide if you want to continue similar marketing initiatives in the future.

CLIENT ACQUISITION

Client acquisition refers to gaining new clients for the business. The primary ways to attract new clients are outlined in this section. When reviewing each of these strategies, think about which ones currently work well for your business. One way to do this is to review the report in your PIMS that shows the source of referral for new clients. Evaluate what's working to attract clients and look for possible areas of opportunity. For example, if the number of new clients who find the practice on the internet isn't high, you may need to invest in digital marketing efforts. Even if you already have marketing initiatives in place for a particular strategy, consider what additional actions you can take for that strategy to bring in even more new clients each month. (See Figure 10.1: Client Acquisition Strategies.)

Location and Hospital Appearance

The practice location may be a principal method of bringing in new clients if the business is conveniently located for pet owners and highly visible to drive-by traffic. Regardless of your location, pay attention to the hospital's exterior appearance. Think about what people see when they drive past the business or into your parking lot. Make sure the outside of the hospital is attractive and projects your desired image. Are trees and bushes trimmed? Are trash receptacles and air conditioner units surrounded by enclosures? Is the property free from debris? Is the façade of the building clean and visually appealing? Is the building well-lit at night? Even businesses with older buildings can create a visually appealing hospital with beautiful landscaping, flower planters, colorful flags, or seasonal displays near the door and clean windows. And don't forget the hospital sign needs to be visible from the street and unobstructed by trees or bushes.

Print Advertising

While it's possible to bring in new clients with print advertising, this is typically an ineffective external marketing strategy for small businesses with limited advertising budgets. Traditional print forms of advertising such as newspaper or magazine ads, yellow page advertising, mass mailings, and newsletters have proven to be of minimal benefit for most veterinary practices in today's world. Print advertising is more likely to work if it's targeted to a specific group of pet owners in the community. If you do spend money on print advertising, be sure to determine the return on investment to see if the strategy was a successful means of client acquisition.

Managers are frequently asked to place ads in community publications such as the high school yearbook, church programs, or local food bank newsletter. Another type of print advertising is to put the logo and hospital name on t-shirts given out for charity events. These forms of advertising don't usually result in gaining a significant number of new clients. But the initiatives often don't cost much and do help promote positive public relations which is good for the business.

Internet

The internet is one of the most effective ways to gain new clients, so the business needs to have a strong digital presence. Most pet owners seeking a new veterinarian go to the internet to explore options for pet care in their area. Therefore, the practice needs to have a website and be visible on social media platforms. Digital marketing is discussed in more detail in the last section of this chapter.

Client Referrals

Most practices have a substantial number of new clients come to the business because an existing client referred them. When a high percentage of new clients are from client referrals, this suggests existing clients are happy and want to spread the word about your practice. Regardless of how many new clients come from personal recommendations, gaining more referrals should be a primary marketing strategy. The best way to drive client referrals is to provide exceptional service and value so existing clients want to recommend the practice to other pet owners. Not only does this strategy increase client acquisition, it also increases client retention.

Additionally, the business can actively strive to increase referrals by simply asking current clients to refer others. Team members can use verbal messages such as "We appreciate your trust and the opportunity to take care of Hannah. Please let your family and friends know about us. We are always looking to add more clients and patients to our family." Another excellent way to increase client referrals is with a referral program that rewards both your existing client and the new client. You might, for example, credit the current client's account $25 (to use for services only) each time they refer a new client and give the new client a complimentary first exam for their pet.

Creating Awareness

An often-overlooked way to attract new clients is to create awareness by having a strong community presence. When pet owners are familiar with the hospital or its veterinarians, they may be more likely to choose the practice for their pets. Practice leaders or the entire team can become active in the community. Managers and practice owners (or other team members) can join Rotary, the Chamber of Commerce, civic or church committees, and local associations. Practice leaders as well as team members can speak at schools or to special interest groups on pet related topics, and volunteer to help with community programs. The practice can also sponsor local activities and charitable events. When sponsoring events, it's always best to set up a display table or request an opportunity to speak at the event. If the practice has a table-top display or booth that features the practice, team members can engage pet owners who attend the event. Have employees working the booth wear shirts with the practice name and attract people with giveaways such as candy, dog treats, magnets, pens, frisbees, and raffle tickets or drawings to win prizes.

Converting Phone Calls to Appointments

Converting phone calls from potential new clients to booked appointments is a valuable strategy for client acquisition. This strategy has gained importance in recent years due to an increase in the call volume from pet owners calling hospitals to inquire about services and the cost of care. The reason for the increase in calls about fees is due to many factors such as a slow economy (at times), financial constraints of pet owners, and the increase in available resources for pet care including low-cost providers. Moreover, today's pet owners often want to explore all their options for pet care.

Historically, calls about fees have been referred to as "phone shoppers." The problem with using this terminology is that it can create a negative impression. Some team members develop a mindset that all these callers care about is money. Most client service representatives (CSRs) don't get excited about handling "phone shopper" calls. In reality, pet owners who call to ask about fees are potential new clients for the business or they may be existing clients who want to know costs and gain more information about the hospital's services. Therefore, better terminology is to change the label from "phone shopper" to "potential new client" or "cost-inquiry" calls.

To convert more phone calls to appointments, managers can set up programs to train team members to use specific communication skills that build trust, engage pet owners, educate callers about pet care services, and showcase the value of being a client at their hospital. According to my analysis of data from mystery shopper calls and that of other companies, there is a significant opportunity to improve phone skills for veterinary teams.

Table 10.1: Client Acquisition Strategies

Strategy	Action Steps
Location and hospital appearance	- Enhance outside building appearance - Ensure outside lighting is sufficient - Make sure hospital signage is visible and well-lit at night - Create visual appeal with landscaping and seasonal displays
Advertising	- Print ads in local publications or at community events - Digital advertising - Content marketing
Internet	- Attractive, up-to-date, engaging website - Increase search engine optimization - Positive online reviews - Social media posts
Client referrals	- Create exceptional client service experiences - Ask for referrals - Client referral program - Network with colleagues and other area businesses
Creating awareness	- Join community associations - Have a presence at community events - Volunteer in the community - Speak to local groups - Provide sponsorship for events
Converting phone calls from potential clients to booked appointments	- Provide phone skills training to team - Always ask for the appointment - Always communicate the value of services

CLIENT ENGAGEMENT

In their book *Human Sigma*, two Principals of Gallup, Joe Fleming and Jim Asplund, define customer engagement as making an emotional connection with people such that they become emotionally satisfied customers.[3] Their research shows customers who are emotionally connected to a business will spend more with the business, be loyal customers, and refer more people to the business. This concept applies equally in veterinary medicine. Clients who are emotionally connected to a practice will say to a friend or co-worker "I wouldn't dream of going anyplace else with my pet."

For veterinary practices, client engagement is about making authentic connections and building trust with pet owners. To attain high levels of client engagement, practices need to be client-focused and adopt a relationship-centered approach to providing care rather than being a doctor-centered hospital. Moreover, teams need to embrace a paradigm of being client-oriented rather than being task-oriented. Team members who focus on building relationships, rather than just completing transactions, can achieve higher levels of client engagement which leads to lead to greater client loyalty, compliance, and referrals.

Building Trust

Everyone wants to do business with people they like and trust. If the relationship between the veterinary team and pet owners isn't built on high levels of trust, pets may not get the care they need. Traditionally, veterinarians have always ranked as one of the most trusted professions.[4] However, this trust should never be taken for granted as clients are trusting the team to provide care for a beloved companion that most consider to be a member of the family. In today's competitive marketplace, people have many choices for where to get pet care. Practice teams should consistently strive to earn and maintain their roles as trusted advisors for pet owners.

When implementing marketing initiatives to increase levels of client engagement, it's advisable to facilitate a team discussion on "building trust." Here are good questions to create dialogue:

- "What does it mean to be trustworthy?"
- "Why do pet owners trust us?"
- "Why wouldn't pet owners trust us?"
- "How do we know if clients trust us?"

Logically, this discussion will lead to team members talking about the importance of providing high quality care, being reliable, and having honest communication with clients. These are all reasons why people trust service providers--medical or otherwise. But equally important, pet owners trust doctors and teams they feel *care* about them and their pet. This is why it's essential that everyone in the practice learns to use specific communication skills that will help them connect emotionally with pet owners.

Team members can use many communication skills to build trust and rapport with pet owners. Certainly, employees need to practice basic skills such as using friendly greetings, addressing clients by their name, and saying thank-you. But teams must go beyond the basics of polite conversation to be able to form emotional connections with pet owners. In the next section, you will learn specific communication skills that are essential to building trust.

Core Client Communication Skills

In human medicine and veterinary medicine alike communication is considered to be a core clinical skill essential to clinical competency.[5] In the book, *Skills for Communicating With Patients*, the authors write that "…. effective communication is essential to high-quality medicine; it improves patient satisfaction, recall, understanding, adherence and outcomes of care."[6] The same can be said of veterinary medicine and in fact significant research shows how better communication leads to greater pet owner satisfaction and improved compliance. The following four core communication skills are the foundation for building trusted relationships and enhancing engagement with pet owners. The value of using these same skills is further explained in the sections of this chapter on client education and increasing client compliance. Managers who implement training programs that afford team members an opportunity to practice core communication skills, are more likely to develop a team that makes it a daily habit of engaging clients. (See Figure 10.2: Team Training Exercises.)

Non-verbal communication

Regardless of what people say, their body language tells a story which makes non-verbal communication just as essential as verbal communication. By observing non-verbal communication, team members can pick up clues about what clients may be feeling and then respond accordingly. Clients who are in a hurry, for example, may repetitively glance at their cellphone or watch, stand instead of sit, or sit on the edge of a chair with folded arms. Unhappy or angry clients may frown, roll their eyes, or stand with hands on their hips. When pet owners are afraid or uncomfortable, they may look down instead of making eye contact, fidget in their chair, or display other nervous behaviors such as clutching their pet.

When a pet has multiple owners, monitor non-verbal communication messages from everyone present to look for any evidence of disharmony or other differences. For example, perhaps one person nods their head in agreement or understanding but their spouse has an expression that conveys skepticism or confusion. To address these mixed messages, ask both owners questions to clarify their thoughts and feelings.

Team members can also be mindful of their own non-verbal communication to ensure it conveys a positive message to clients. Eye-contact is a key component of non-verbal communication and critical to making connections with people. This is why it's vital to look at pet owners when they're talking and minimize time spent looking at a computer during exam room conversations. Other positive non-verbal communications such as smiling, nodding of the head, and leaning slightly toward the client also demonstrate an interest in clients and a desire to help them.

Open-ended questions

People can answer a close-ended question with a "yes", "no" or a one-word response so it doesn't always promote dialogue. On the other hand, open-ended questions invite the other person to share information which is why this is one of the best ways to engage pet owners. Veterinary teams routinely ask pet owners many close-ended questions such as "How old is Chloe?" or "Has your address changed?" These are relevant questions, but don't serve to build trust and make connections with clients.

Open-ended questions help team members express a genuine interest in the client and their pet. Moreover, open-ended questions encourage dialogue which helps team members develop more meaningful relationships with clients. Examples of open-ended questions used to build trust and rapport include:

- "What toys does Sadie like to play with?"
- "What do you have planned for the holidays?"
- "Tell me how your daughter is doing in soccer."
- "How did you decide to get a Papillon?"
- "Tell me more about your concerns."

Open-ended questions also support the veterinary team in their efforts to understand clients and uncover what's important to them for their pet's healthcare which helps build trust. Examples of these open-ended questions include:

- "How did you decide to give this supplement?"
- "Tell me about Jake's lifestyle and how you spend time together."
- "What's important to you for Scooter's well-being and dental health?"
- "What do you think about Charlie's response to treatment?"
- "Tell me what's most important to you for Hannah's diet."

Reflective listening

Reflective listening is a communication skill often used to ensure a clear understanding of what pet owners have told the team about their pet. In this case, team members repeat back to the client what they heard or summarize the client's words. For example, the veterinarian may say "So, if I understand correctly, Jake stopped eating yesterday, vomited twice this morning, and doesn't seem to be feeling well." This type of reflective listening statement invites the client to affirm the doctor has understood them correctly. If the doctor didn't understand or made an erroneous assumption, the client has an opportunity to clarify the information.

In addition, reflective listening statements can be used to invite clients to share more information about the pet as well as their thoughts, feelings, and needs. In this instance, reflective listening helps clients feel heard and hopefully more comfortable sharing their feelings. This leads to stronger, trusted relationships between team members and clients. Examples of these types of reflective listening statements include:

- "I'm hearing you say that you think Oliver's quality of life is not good, is that correct?"
- "I understand that you have some budget constraints for what you can spend today."
- "If I am hearing you correctly, it sounds like you aren't sure which treatment option is best for Lindsey?"
- "It sounds like you have concerns about how you and your husband will take care of Ginger."
- "I sense you aren't sure whether to proceed with chemotherapy for Violet."

Figure 10.1: Team Training Exercises

> **Client Communications Training: Enhancing Client Engagement**
>
> Paired or group exercises:
>
> **1. Asking clients open-ended questions**
>
> Purpose: For team members to learn the value of using open-ended questions to build trust and rapport with clients. This exercise helps employees understand the difference between close-ended and open-ended questions. By practicing asking open-ended questions, team members gain insight about how they can use these questions to learn more information and connect with pet owners.
>
> Description: Ideally, pair team members together who don't know each other well for this exercise. Start the exercise by having each team member ask their co-worker an open-ended question to get to know the other person better. Examples: "Tell me about your last vacation" or "How do you like to spend your spare time?" Allow no more than two minutes for this exercise so everyone understands asking open-ended questions doesn't take substantially more time than close-ended questions.
>
> Debrief as a team: Share what questions participants asked each other and what they learned about their co-worker. Verify that questions were truly open-ended questions. Sometimes team members ask close-ended questions such as "How many pets do you have?" Their co-worker may tell them about all their pets because they want to engage in dialogue. However, this is a closed-ended question that could be answered with a one-word response. There isn't anything wrong with asking closed-ended questions, but the team needs to appreciate that open-ended questions are more engaging.
>
> Next ask participants to ask each other an open-ended question that they might ask a client. Examples: "What kind of activities does Gidget like?" or "Tell me a little bit about Cooper's lifestyle."
>
> Debrief again as a team to see what interesting questions the team came up with. In addition, brainstorm relevant questions to ask new clients or those clients team members don't know well. This is much harder than asking questions of an established client. Examples: "Why did you name your cat Penelope?" or "How did you decide to choose our practice?"
>
> **2. Understanding nonverbal communications**
>
> Purpose: Clients' body language often conveys information about their thoughts and feelings. Team members who are mindful of observing clients' non-verbal communication and know how to respond can build stronger connections with pet owners. This exercise helps team members understand the value of being aware of nonverbal communication and effective ways to connect with clients who may be exhibiting emotions such as anger, frustration, fear, concern, sadness, or grief.

Figure 10.2: Team Training Exercises (continued)

> Description: Have team members work in pairs or as a small group. Each team member takes a turn stating a client's non-verbal communication they might observe. Their partner or another member of the group then states what message they think is conveyed by the non-verbal and how they would respond to the client.
>
> Example: One team member says they observe non-verbal communication of a client looking at a cell phone. Their co-worker responds that the message conveyed by the client might be that they're bored, disinterested, in a hurry, or waiting on an important message. An excellent response to the client would be to say "Mrs. Smith, I noticed you looking at your cell phone. Do you need some time to take care of your messages or are you in a hurry?" By responding to the non-verbal message, the team member confirms the client's feelings and hopefully politely conveys the need to engage in dialogue about their pet.

Empathy statements

Empathy can be defined as the ability to sense and understand another person's emotions and to imagine what someone else might be thinking or feeling. Sympathy on the other hand is expressing pity or feeling bad for someone. Renowned author, Brené Brown, offers an excellent explanation of the difference between these two communications by explaining that "empathy fuels connection" while "sympathy drives disconnections".[7] Empathy statements can be used by team members to acknowledge the client's perspective, emotions, and feelings. Expressing empathy helps people feel heard and bonds them to the hospital team. Not only does empathy lead to enhanced client engagement and loyalty but also greater client compliance and better medical outcomes. When people's needs are met, they are more open to working with the healthcare team to get their pet's needs met.

Empathy involves being fully present with the other person and a willingness to be vulnerable to reach a deeper connection. You don't have to feel the same emotion as the client feels or have experienced their feelings to express empathy. Striving to appreciate someone's predicament or feelings is what is important as well as supportively communicating that understanding to the person. Be mindful to slow down when expressing empathy. All too often, team members try to fix problems or jump too quickly to explanations without spending enough time expressing empathy. To avoid this pitfall, team members can practice making eye contact and pausing after saying an empathy statement.

It's a common tendency for team members to relate their personal experiences with pet illness. Be careful when expressing shared feelings because it can draw attention away from the client. Pet owners want to focus on their pet and may feel their situation is uniquely different. If a team member has a pet with a similar medical condition or has been in the same situation, it may be helpful to convey this to the client but keep the reference short with a comment such as "I had a Papillon with heart failure several years ago. She was on six different medications, and I remember feeling frustrated and sad at times."

Bear in mind that many people naturally tend to express sympathy rather than empathy. Remember sympathy is feeling sorry for someone. Here are examples:

- "I'm so sorry to hear you were laid off. I'm sure you'll find a new job."
- "That's too bad. At least you're coping with everything."
- "I'm sorry about your situation. I'm sure things will get better soon."

By contrast, empathy statements are more personal, convey a deeper level of understanding, and avoid pity. Here are examples of empathy statements:

- "I can sense that you are worried about Sophie."
- "I can see this is a difficult time for you. I'm here for you."
- "I can imagine it was scary to go through that experience."
- "It sounds like you've done everything you could for Chloe."
- "I appreciate you weren't expecting this diagnosis or expense to treat Miranda's condition."

CLIENT EDUCATION

Client education is an indispensable component of internal marketing because if pet owners don't understand their pet's health status and medical conditions, they may not say "yes" to pet care recommendations. Sometimes pet owners lack basic knowledge about preventive care such as the need for annual heartworm and intestinal parasite testing. Clients may also have read or heard false information about pet care which leads them to forego veterinary visits and decline treatment plans. Additionally, clients may view recommendations as a sales pitch if team members don't fully educate them about why *their* pet needs care. To overcome the barriers presented by these scenarios, it's imperative teams strive to form a partnership with pet owners and provide more personalized client education.

Partnering with Clients

Pet owners appreciate a collaborative approach to client education where they're brought into the conversation about their pet's healthcare. With this method of client education, the veterinary team encourages dialogue with pet owners which helps them feel heard and empowered. The concept is to form a partnership and is often referred to as a shared decision-making model for healthcare whereby medical professionals work together with patients (or clients) to make medical decisions.[8] Shared decision-making in veterinary medicine supports engaging pet owners in a collaborative process so they can make medical care decisions and choose a treatment plan that is best for their pet and family. It involves serving as a guide for our clients rather than only adopting a paternalistic approach of telling clients "This is what you need to do" or "This is what I recommend." The goal of shared decision-making is to achieve better patient outcomes.

Since client education is such an integral part of veterinary medicine, it's easy for veterinarians in particular to adopt a paternalistic approach to communication that conveys "I know best." Some clients may not be open to hearing what doctors have to say if they don't feel heard or if they have different ideas about their pet's medical care. The key to partnering with pet owners is for team members to avoid lecturing clients and instead practice asking questions that promote discussion and shared understanding.

To ensure team members partner with clients, follow the communication paradigm of "connect before you convince." This is especially important when pet owners have limited knowledge or faulty beliefs about medical topics. Open-ended questions are the best way to connect with pet owners and assess what they know about their pet's health and medical condition. Here are examples:

- "Tell me what you know about heart failure in dogs."
- "What have you heard about treating cats with diabetes?"
- "Tell me what you've read about the best diet to feed Daisy."
- "May I give you some information on orthopedic problems that are common for dachshunds?"
- "Would you be open to discussing how we can best meet Bella's nutritional needs and a few diet options?"

These questions show respect for the client's views, bring the client into the conversation, and ask for permission to educate rather than launching into what may be perceived as a lecture and fall on deaf ears. Open-ended questions also help team members avoid making assumptions about what pet owners know so they can better tailor client education messages and increase efficiency during appointments.

Improving Client Education Messages

Client education needs to be accurate and consistent which means everyone on the team should be trained to convey the same information. Otherwise, people may hear different messages from different team members. When this happens, pet owners may be confused, and trust starts to breakdown. Imagine how a pet owner might feel if a team member tells them they don't need to worry about heartworm prevention in the winter and later they hear about the importance of year-round protection. They may feel uneasy about the quality and consistency of care at the hospital.

It's also important for client education to be comprehensive meaning it should provide sufficient details about all aspects of the pet's physical exam, medical condition, and treatment options. The best way to educate pet owners during their pet's physical exam is to communicate every action. Clients understand what happens during auscultation of their pet's heart but may have no idea what is going on when doctors palpate the pet's lymph nodes and abdomen. This is why it's important to narrate the physical exam, so clients know what is being examined and why. Likewise, be sure to convey thorough information when discussing the pet's illness and possible treatments. While clients appreciate easy to understand lay terms, they also want meaningful information about their pet's condition and prognosis. Remember, today's pet parents are knowledgeable and have easy access to information on the internet

Client education is more meaningful for clients if it's tailored specifically for *their* pet. Pet-specific care in its entirety is the subject of the book, *Pet Specific Care for the Veterinary Team* by Dr. Lowell Ackerman.[9] Dr. Ackerman defines pet specific care as, "veterinary care tailored to individual pets based on their risk of disease and their likely response to intervention. At its core, pet-specific care focuses on prevention, early detection and evidence-based management using a pet's individual risk factors and circumstances to determine the best course of action."[10]

To engage in pet specific client education, avoid talking in generalities about pet care and instead convey personalized education messages. One way to do this is to reference the pet's lifestyle, age, breed, and risk factors. Don't forget to use the pet's name instead of using phrases such as "all dogs", "our pets", or "outdoor cats." For example, let's say Ms. Smith brings in Molly, her overweight, nine-year old dachshund that spends most of the time on the couch. While it's true all dogs should be on year-round heartworm prevention, Ms. Smith really just cares about what Molly needs. She may not perceive the need for heartworm or flea prevention since her beloved companion spends limited time outdoors. In this instance, team members can address specifically why Molly needs these preventive care products rather than talking about all dogs or Ms. Smith may be unconvinced.

Use of Visual Tools

Using a visual aid adds value to the client education process because it can help improve clients' understanding of their pet's medical condition, healthcare needs, and treatment recommendations. Visual tools enhance the retention of information and can make client education more engaging for pet owners. In part this happens because visual aids trigger both the auditory and visual senses of a person. Studies show the use of visuals helps people better comprehend and remember information.[11]

Teams can use many visual aids including brochures, client handouts, graphs, charts, drawings, photos, anatomical models, radiographs, lab work results, and videos. Ideally, some type of visual tool should be used for every appointment unless it is a medical progress exam. Here are specific examples of how to use visual aids for client education:

- Show a client ear mites or demodectic mange mites under the microscope
- Use an anatomical model of an ear when talking about otitis externa and how to clean ears
- Show a client a graph that depicts the trend for their cat's kidney function lab values
- Use the body condition scoring chart when discussing obesity; have clients identify which picture looks like their pet
- Review videos with a client to determine if their dog is exhibiting a reverse sneeze or a cough
- Show a client before and after photos of pets that have had dental procedures to demonstrate the value of these services

INCREASING CLIENT COMPLIANCE

Broadly, client compliance refers to whether pet owners say yes to recommendations for preventive care as well as medical, dental, and surgical treatment plans. Historically, multiple veterinary organizations, companies, and individual hospitals have reported lower than desired rates of client compliance for preventive care services and products such as annual physical exams, parasite testing, flea/tick/heartworm preventives, dentistry procedures and blood work. Client compliance rates for sick pets that need care is harder to track and extremely variable from practice to practice.

AAHA published a study on compliance in 2003 called The Path to High-Quality Care.[12] The 2009 AAHA Compliance Follow-Up Study reported rates of compliance compared to their 2003 study.[13] The report showed variable rates of compliance for preventive care services. Two examples of low compliance in 2009 were that only 51% of dogs were on heartworm preventive and only 38% of animals with a need for dentals received care. In 2019, a study by Ceva Animal Health found that only 25% of dogs were receiving heartworm prevention regularly and that 27% of the dog owners thought they were giving heartworm prevention, but they were only giving flea and tick prevention.[14]

The 2011 Bayer Veterinary Care Usage Study evaluated reasons for the disturbing trend of a decline in patient visits for veterinary practices.[15] It identified the following contributing factors to whether pet owners come in for routine preventive care and whether they say yes to recommendations: state of the economy, cost of care, stress of visits, increased usage of the Web to learn about pet health, expansion of veterinary services including easy access to lower cost options, and lack of understanding or perception of the value of services.

Increasing client compliance should be a primary marketing initiative since it is perhaps the greatest opportunity to increase service and product utilization and thus increase revenues. However, managers often find this to be a frustrating marketing strategy because they receive pushback from team members who are weary of hearing "no" or "not now" from pet owners. Moreover, practice teams may feel limited in what they can do to improve compliance. To enhance the success of marketing initiatives aimed at increasing client compliance, first measure the current rates of compliance. Then after launching a marketing effort, monitor monthly KPIs. Practices can calculate compliance rates to some extent by evaluating PIMS reports but this process can be tedious and time-consuming. Alternatively, managers can find outside companies that place a data extraction tool on the server. The company extracts and analyzes data to present practices with key metrics. Recognize that it may take months of sustained team efforts to increase compliance rates.

In the rest of this section, we look at six ways practices can increase client compliance. Focus on implementing only a few changes at a time. This makes it easier to know what's working well to improve compliance. It also helps set your team up for success since they are the ones to execute your marketing plans. Team members are more likely to affect change if they can focus on using only one or two communications skills at a time.

Reminder Systems

First and foremost, an effective reminder system is necessary to improve client compliance. People rely on their personal healthcare providers and many other companies to remind them when it's time to schedule appointments. Likewise, clients rely on the veterinary practice to let them know when their pets are due for routine preventive healthcare. Since pet owners don't perceive a sense of urgency to schedule preventive care appointments, it's imperative that practices remind them when their pet is due for healthcare services and products.

Sending out at least 3 reminders for routine preventive care is considered a best practice. Pet owners should receive a combination of regular mail postcards, emails, text messages, push notifications, and phone calls taking into consideration client preferences. Some practices have eliminated mailed postcards since many clients prefer digital reminders. In addition to sending reminders for preventive care such as annual exams, vaccines and parasite testing, hospitals can increase compliance by establishing patient reminders for lab panels, medical progress exams, and refills for all medications, therapeutic diets and flea, tick, and heartworm preventives.

Communicating Value

Since team members often feel they regularly communicate the value of services to pet owners, managers may want to facilitate dialogue on the question of "how can we *better* communicate the value of our services and products?" This helps to achieve buy-in on the need to implement marketing initiatives in this area. Remind everyone that learning communications to enhance clients' understanding about the value of services helps them fulfill their roles as trusted advisors for pet owners. The reward of using specific communication skills to increase compliance is more pets care get care they deserve.

Communicating the value of veterinary services begins with communicating the value of the physical exam and consultation. The first opportunity to do this usually occurs when pet owners call to inquire about a preventive care exam or an exam for a sick pet. Team members who answer phones should communicate the value of the "office call" (or whatever terminology the practice uses) when quoting fees. They might say, "Our doctors will do a comprehensive examination of Lola to be sure she is healthy. This includes checking her out from the tip of her nose to the end of her tail. They will also discuss all aspects of her healthcare and answer any questions you may have." Additionally, remember to always convey the value of the physical exam if the client wasn't present for the doctor's exam. Don't make the mistake of only saying "I examined Lola and she looks great" or "Dr. Smith examined Lola, and everything was fine." Instead describe specific findings of the entire exam even if it was normal so the client can fully appreciate the value of having their pet examined by a veterinarian.

Team members can make similar statements when talking to pet owners about other services. Rather than just quoting fees or telling clients what their pet is due for, focus on communicating the value of the services. Don't assume pet owners are knowledgeable about basic preventive pet care. A team member might say "Rusty is due for his distemper-parvo immunization today. We use a safe vaccine that has been proven to offer protection against these two most common, life-threatening viral diseases. He won't need another booster for three years."

Likewise, if Rusty had an ear infection, the technician or assistant might say "Dr. Taylor would like to further evaluate Rusty's ear infection by performing an otic cytology. [explain the procedure] This test determines what type of infection is present, how severe it is, and gives Dr. Taylor the information she needs to prescribe the best medication for Rusty. This is important because we want Rusty to feel better as soon as possible and eliminate his infection."

Making Clear Recommendations

If pet owners aren't clear on what action to take, they may decline or defer recommendations. And in many instances, it may not be obvious when clients have said "no." Clients may leave the hospital without purchasing flea, tick, or heartworm preventives. They may not purchase a recommended therapeutic diet. They may not schedule a medical progress exam, dentistry procedure, or mass removal that was discussed. When this happens, it's often because the client didn't clearly understand the recommendation or is confused about their different options.

Strive to eliminate vague, tentative language when making recommendations. One study found clients were seven times more likely to agree to a recommendation for dentistry or surgery if they received a clear recommendation rather than one that was ambiguous from the veterinarian.[16] Examples of ambiguous language include phrases such as "it would be a good idea to get Gretchen's teeth cleaned,", "you should probably see about getting Hannah's teeth cleaned" or "we ought to get Chloe's teeth cleaned when you can." There isn't a call to action or a sense of urgency with these statements. The language makes it sound like dentistry is simply an option for consideration rather than a need for the patient to receive the best care. To establish need and next steps, a veterinarian can say, "Due to Molly's grade III periodontal disease and the probability that she is experiencing some discomfort, I recommend you schedule her oral assessment, treatment and prevention (oral ATP) as soon as possible. Jill will help you get her appointment set up."

In addition to establishing a timeline for care, recommendations should convey clarity in terms of which treatment is most beneficial for the patient. Unfortunately, exam room observations reveal that sometimes veterinarians give clients a confusing list of multiple alternatives for treatment. It might sound like this: "We could do….", "sometimes we do…..", "you could take antibiotics…..", "we can try medication and see if that helps", "I'm thinking doing x-rays and lab testing would be helpful." Aside from tentative language used in these statements, the primary problem is the lack of clarity regarding which treatment plan may be best for the patient.

Being transparent about various treatment options is an essential component of the shared decision-making model. However, clients still need an explanation of the benefits (or drawbacks) of different treatment plans. If pet owners are left to believe two or three treatment options are equally beneficial, they'll likely gravitate towards the least expensive and least scary plan. Since clients generally don't have the medical knowledge to decide which treatment or products are best, they need the veterinary team to provide guidance. For example, for a vomiting patient, the veterinarian might say "The benefit of laboratory testing is we will gain valuable information that will help us know how to best treat Sophie. The risk of not doing the testing is that we may not uncover whether she is dehydrated or has evidence of pancreatitis."

Teams also need to convey clear recommendations for products such as preventives, supplements, therapeutic diets, ear cleaners, and shampoos. Clients who leave without purchasing products usually do so because they either weren't convinced of the value of the product, think they can purchase it online for less, or are confused because they were presented with too many options. To enhance compliance for product sales, here are best practices:

- Make a *specific* recommendation that includes the brand name of the product. Without a specific brand name, clients are left to assume any product they buy on the internet is fine.
- Avoid confusion by giving clients as few options as possible. When discussing more than one product, offer guidance on which one is best based on the different features.

- Clearly communicate specific benefits about how the product will help the pet. For example, a weight loss diet helps the pet lose weight but what is the benefit? Be sure to discuss benefits such as improved mobility, less pain, reduced chance of other medical problems and prolonged life span.

When making recommendations, avoid making assumptions about what pet owners want or whether they can afford to pay for treatment. Instead, base recommendations on patient advocacy. Of course, the practice should have as many options in place as possible to help clients afford care.

Talking About Money

Veterinary care can be expensive and only a small percentage of pet owners have pet insurance. According to AVMA data, the average annual household income for almost 50% of pet owners is less than $60,000 per year.[17] Pet owners in all income brackets may have limited funds for pet care and it's safe to say, all clients appreciate having the ability to spread out the cost of care. In addition to accepting credit cards, practices can use an array of payment solutions including pet insurance, third-party payment plans, preventive care plans, and managed payment plans.

Regardless of the state of the economy or the financial means of clients, it makes sense for practice teams to be well-trained to have honest, supportive conversations with pet owners about fees. Rather than waiting for clients to ask about payment options, train your team to proactively discuss fees and payments. They can say "Mr. Jones, I know these were unexpected services for Charlie. We do have several payment solutions. Would you like me to review those with you now?"

Forward Booking

Dentists and physicians embraced forward booking many years ago. Rarely do we leave their offices without scheduling our next appointment. Veterinary practices can implement the same protocol. Regardless of whether a pet is due to be seen again in two days, two months or a year, set up the next appointment before the client leaves the hospital. Forward booking increases compliance because clients are more likely to come back when their pet needs care if they have a booked appointment. One way to measure the effectiveness of forward booking is to look at the hospital client visitation rate which is a measure of how often active clients visit the practice.

Make is a standard hospital protocol to proactively ask for the appointment and use communication skills that convey the value of the next exam. Unfortunately, team members often use tentative language by saying "Did you want to schedule your next appointment?" This is a closed-ended question that clients can easily respond to with "Not now, I'll just call you back." A better approach is to use the doctor's name, express the need for the appointment, convey value. and offer specific times. Here is an example:

> "Dr. Carlson needs to examine Max's skin and ears again in 2 weeks. She'll assess his response to treatment which is important to make sure the infection has resolved and determine if he needs more antibiotics. Is this same time, Wednesday at 3pm good for you that week? Of course, we will send you reminders prior to Max's appointment."

Handling Angry Clients

One of the biggest frustrations and challenges in veterinary medicine is dealing with angry clients. Teams trained to respond positively to angry pet owners can help increase compliance. The first step when interacting with angry clients is to maintain a calm demeanor and actively listen. Team members' body language and facial expressions should convey interest and a genuine desire to help. As stated earlier, this includes leaning forward slightly, nodding, and maintaining eye contact.

Next, seek to understand why a pet owner is angry. Anger is often a secondary emotion. Sometimes people use anger as a shield or protective mechanism when they're experiencing more painful emotions such as fear, sadness, and grief. In these instances, clients may display anger even though their primary feeling is that they're scared or sad about their pet's condition. Understanding this concept can make it easier to remember to respond to irate clients with compassion.

To identify if there is an underlying emotion triggering anger, listen to clients and allow them to thoroughly explain their frustrations. Avoid interrupting pet owners, as this may exacerbate their anger. Consider if a client has valid complaints. Observe whether they're clearly under stress or afraid they may not be able to afford care. Look for evidence that a client has anticipatory grief about the loss of a pet. The best way to further explore reasons why a client might be distressed is to ask open-ended questions. Open-ended questions help teams avoid assumptions and learn more about what clients might be feeling.

Here are examples of good questions to ask:
- "Are you worried that Merlin might not do well with the treatment?"
- "Ms. Martin, I sense you're concerned. How can I help?"

- "I understand you're upset that Dr. Fowler isn't available. Is there anything else?"

Seek to connect with angry pet owners regardless of why they're emotional. Clients may be concerned that they can't afford treatment, afraid of how family members will react to their decisions, or afraid their pet is going to die. Strive to reassure clients and validate their emotions. Team members can express empathy and offer reassurance with statements such as:

- "I realize this is a difficult time for you."
- "I know this is upsetting and I understand you're angry."
- "I know you weren't expecting this outcome today and how much Red means to you."
- "We know Maggie is a special member of your family and how much you love her. We're going to do everything we can to help her."

BUILDING CLIENT LOYALTY AND MEETING CLIENT'S NEEDS

Client retention is defined as the ability of a practice to retain clients, meaning they continue to purchase services and products from the practice. But just because businesses retain clients doesn't necessarily mean they're loyal. Pet owners may continue to visit a veterinary hospital because it's conveniently located and provides the veterinary services their pet needs. But they may not feel bonded to the practice if the client experience isn't exceptional or if they determine their needs can easily be met from another practice.

The goal for veterinary practices is to not only have high levels of client retention but more importantly to have high levels of client loyalty. Loyal clients wouldn't dream of taking their pets somewhere else and they generally refer other pet owners to the practice. To build client loyalty, evaluate how well your business is doing meeting the needs of clients. Begin by thinking about what pet owners in your community want from a veterinary provider. This may vary depending on the demographics of the area. Clients in an urban setting, for example, may have different needs and place value on different services than pet owners in a suburban area with many retirees.

Human-Animal Bond

Regardless of demographics, most pet owners seek veterinary care because of the human-animal bond. The average pet owner considers their pet a member of the family and wants access to high quality veterinary care. They also desire a trusted relationship. Pet owners want to take their pet to a hospital where the team clearly cares about their pet and the bond they share with their companion.

Interestingly, surveys and research show pet owners, especially those from younger generations, consider a pet's diet, exercise, play and emotional well-being as part of preventive care.[18] Therefore, teams are wise to discuss all aspects of the pet's life with clients. Not only do these conversations reveal valuable information about the pet's health, but this holistic approach also reinforces the role of the veterinary team as trusted advisors.

As stated by the AVMA, the role of veterinarians in the human-animal bond is to maximize the beneficial relationship between people and pets by promoting health and well-being of both.[19] One of the ways veterinarians do this is through collaborative care partnerships between primary care veterinarians and veterinary specialists. While not every client can afford or desires specialty care, they appreciate being informed about the availability and benefits of specialized veterinary medicine.

Generational Differences

In 2019, the Pew Research Center reported that according to population estimates from the U.S. Census Bureau, millennials had surpassed baby boomers as the nation's largest living adult generation.[20] They define millennials as ages 23 to 38 in 2019 and boomers as ages 55 to 73. They also reported that Generation X, defined as ages 39 to 54 were projected to pass the boomers in population by 2028. Multiple organizations have reported that millennials, also known as Generation Y, are now the primary pet-owning demographic. Both millennials and the newest generation called Generation Z (born between 1995 and 2015), have high rates of pet ownership. Of course, practices also have clients who are traditionalists (born between 1925-1945).

Veterinary practice teams that focus on meeting the needs of pet parents of all generations will best ensure the long-term success of the business. When considering how to best meet the needs of clients and build loyalty, remember to think about what pet owners value. Pet parents from all generations value feeling connected to a trusted advisor that cares about them and their pet. Likewise, pet owners appreciate a personalized, memorable client experience. Therefore, marketing initiatives that focus on improving client engagement and client education universally cater to the needs of all pet owners.

Generally speaking, younger generations prefer to stay in touch with veterinary practices via texts, mobile applications, and digital platforms. On the other hand, older generations may prefer mailed reminders, personal phone calls and emails. But be cautious not to stereotype generations or make assumptions about what type of communications they desire. Rather, adapt communication methods to the preferences of each pet owner. It may be true that some older clients prefer phone calls to texts, but this isn't universally the case. There are many boomers who do most of their communication via texts rather than email. Increasingly older generations have embraced using smartphones, social media, and mobile apps. (See figures 10.2 and 10.3 on generational differences.)[21]

Figure 10.2: Social Media Usage by Generation in the United States, 2019

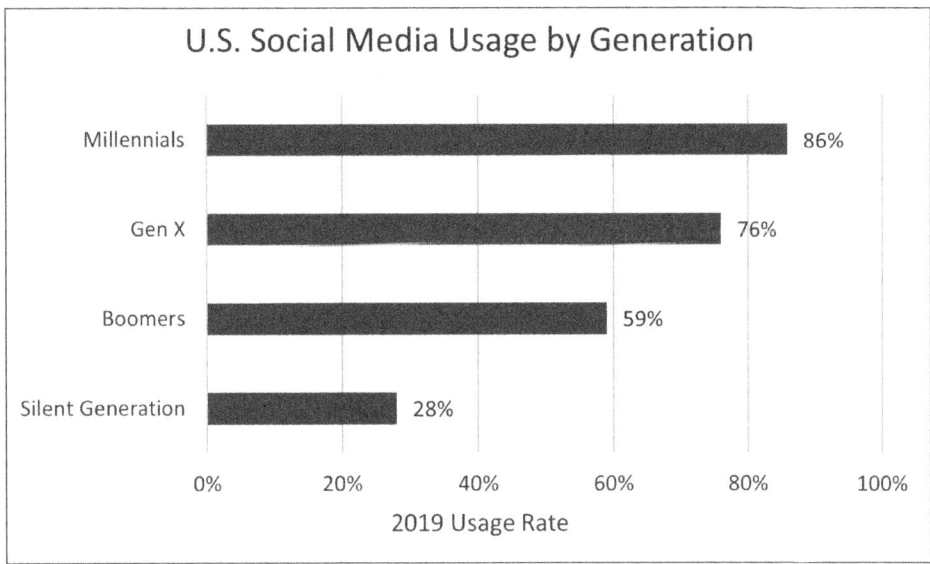

Source: Adapted from Pew Research Center data, Millennials stand out for their technology use, but older generations also embrace digital life by Emily A. Vogels, https://www.pewresearch.org/fact-tank/2019/09/09/us-generations-technology-use/, September 9, 2019.

It's noteworthy that research shows millennials place significant importance on values and making a difference in the world. They prefer doing business with companies that share their values. This is one of many reasons why it's ideal to communicate the core values of the practice and share your love of veterinary medicine as well as any involvement the practice has in helping the community. Younger generations also have a greater desire to stay connected to companies they do business with. Therefore, it's beneficial to consider how to stay in touch and meet the needs of pet parents before, during, and after appointments.

Figure 10.3: Facebook Usage by Generation in the United States, 2012 to 2019

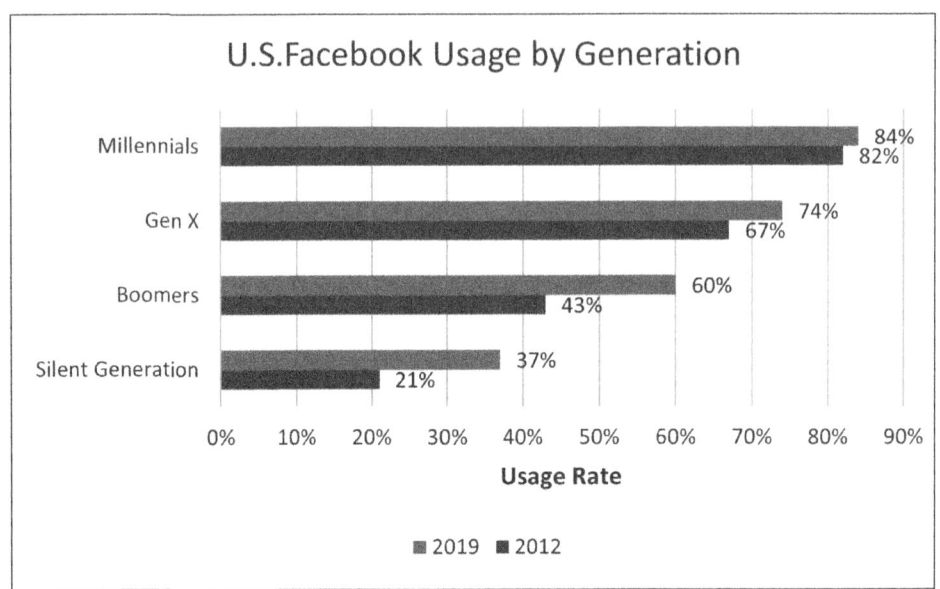

Source: Adapted from Pew Research Center data, Millennials stand out for their technology use, but older generations also embrace digital life by Emily A. Vogels, https://www.pewresearch.org/fact-tank/2019/09/09/us-generations-technology-use/, *September 9, 2019.*

Convenient, Personalized Service

Today's consumers want convenience which is why online shopping and home delivery options are so popular. Companies like Amazon, Blue Apron, Uber, Nordstrom, and Netflix are successful, in part, because they offer consumers the convenience they crave. People also have a strong desire for customized service. Nordstrom has personal stylists and Amazon's Alexa reminds you when you may want to re-order products. Amazon also lets you create lists and pet profiles on its site. Netflix emails you when they add a show or movie you might. Another example of personalized, convenient service is car dealerships that provide free pick-up and delivery service for car maintenance.

Since people have grown accustomed to increased accessibility to services and products, look for ways to increase convenience for pet owners. Many practices have moved to exam room checkout procedures which clients appreciate since it's more comfortable and easier to have private conversations about payment options. Likewise, it's a better experience for clients who might have to juggle multiple pets, kids, purses, and take-home medications if they check out at the front desk. Another way to offer convenience that practices became aware of because of the 2020 COVID-19 pandemic is curbside care. While this isn't a desirable business model to replace in in-person visits, it can work well to accommodate clients who just want to pick up prescriptions or who have special needs such as limited mobility. (For more ideas, see textbox, "Ways to Provide Convenient Service to Clients.")

> **WAYS TO PROVIDE CONVENIENT SERVICE TO CLIENTS**
> - Hospital online pharmacy
> - Exam room check-out procedures
> - Provide boarding and grooming services
> - Curbside or drive-through service
> - Home delivery of prescriptions and pet food
> - Day admissions for patient care
> - Extended hours during the week and/or weekend hours
> - Access to trusted pet sitters
> - Access to pet day care, puppy/kitten socialization, and dog training services
> - Mobile services such as house calls or pick-up and delivery of patients
> - Access to client liaisons to ask questions and get patient status updates

Given the busy lifestyles and demands of clients, evaluate whether it' easy for pet owners to do business with the practice. In his book, *The Convenience Revolution*, Shep Hyken, writes that the primary principle of the customer experience is to reduce friction.[22] Basically, friction is anything that doesn't go well from the customer's perspective. Think about what pet owners want and any pain points during the client service experience at your hospital. One obvious example is appointment wait times. Clients tend to become frustrated if there is a lengthy check-in procedure when dropping off pets for surgery, medical treatment, boarding, or grooming. (See Chapter 8 for action steps on how to increase operational efficiency.) Other times when pet owners might experience friction occur when they call and are put on hold or when they have to take time out of their day to pick up medications.

Practices can leverage technology to help pet owners stay connected to the practice, save time, and provide convenient, customized service. The vast majority of today's pet parents are busy and spend a considerable amount of time on their smartphones or other mobile devices such as tablets, laptop computers, and smart watches. When evaluating technology solutions, be sure to consider whether it helps clients and helps pets get care they deserve. (See textbox, "Technology Solutions Desired by Pet Owners.")

TECHNOLOGY SOLUTIONS DESIRED BY PET OWNERS

- 24/7 access to online appointment scheduling
- Two-way texting with the hospital team
- Digital access to the pet's veterinary medical records
- Text reminders for appointments and patient care
- Apps that track medication usage and pet activity levels
- Online forms to complete new client information and the patient's history
- A telehealth approach or telemedicine so pet owners can video chat, text, or email with a veterinarian
- Text messages about patient care updates, food or prescription refill requests, and targeted messages
- Contactless payment via links to payment options such as Google pay, Apple pay, Paypal, hospital apps or third-party plans

---

Client loyalty programs

Customer loyalty programs are a proven marketing tool to increase customer retention. They're popular for businesses such as airlines, hotels, car rental agencies, restaurants, and many other retailers. Companies endeavor to build loyalty by rewarding their most frequent customers with cash, discounts, free services or products, or other value-added services and products. Client loyalty programs in veterinary medicine work the same way. Pet owners may be more bonded to a practice that offers some type of perks. Often veterinary loyalty programs offer clients cash rewards based on how much they spend.

Since people are generally tied to their cell phones, the practice may want to use a client loyalty program that is accessed via a mobile app. Multiple veterinary marketing companies offer mobile apps branded to the practice that include customizable client loyalty programs as one of the features. Often these companies have case studies or customer testimonials on their websites showing how loyalty programs have increased pet owner spending at the hospital.

DIGITAL MARKETING

Hubspot, a company specializing in helping businesses grow, defines digital marketing as follows:

"Digital marketing encompasses all marketing efforts that use an electronic device or the internet. Businesses leverage digital channels such as search engines, social media, email, and other websites to connect with current and prospective customers."[23] In this section, we cover four relevant aspects of digital marketing for veterinary practices.

Websites and Search Engine Optimization

The practice website is a primary marketing strategy for any veterinary business. Pet owners turn to the internet to find pet care information, locate veterinary providers in their area, and read more about a hospital. For the practice website to enhance client acquisition and retention, it must be easily found when people type key words in their internet browser. The average person doesn't look at websites that don't show up on the first page of an internet search which is why the practice website needs to have good search engine optimization (SEO).

Entire books are written on SEO but simply defined it's the process of making changes to a website or webpage so it's more visible and thus ranks higher in a search engine's un-paid ("organic") search results. The higher the ranking on the search results page, the more visitors to the site. To test the SEO for your business, type key words and phrases into an internet browser such as Microsoft Edge, Google Chrome, Mozilla Firefox, or Apple's Safari. This might include "animal hospital near me", "veterinary clinic", and "pet hospital". Does your hospital show up in the top 5 listings or at least on the first page of the search? If not, then the practice website can benefit from efforts to improve SEO.

Enhancing SEO begins by having a website professionally designed by experts that understand how to maximize SEO. It may also be beneficial to hire a marketing company to help the practice achieve higher rankings. Don't forget that with the increase in usage of mobile devices, it's important to make sure the practice website is easy to navigate on a mobile device. You can use this website to test whether your website is mobile friendly: https://search.google.com/test/mobile-friendly.

Once pet owners reach the practice website, they need to be able to easily find information such as the hospital phone number, online forms, and pertinent details about the business. The two most frequently visited pages are the Home page and the About Us page. These pages should be visually appealing with professional, high-quality photos. Be sure to include photos of the doctors along with their bios and be careful to avoid the use of stock photos that may appear on multiple veterinary practice websites. Likewise, try to use real-life photos of the hospital and the team rather than stock images. There are many website design and marketing companies that build beautiful, contemporary websites that promote the human-animal bond and help showcase why the pet owner should choose the practice.

Ads and Content Marketing

Google Ads and Facebook Ads are the two most popular companies for paid search, also known as pay-per-click (PPC) advertising platforms. Google Ads work with SEO to increase the business's ranking on the search engine ranking page (SERP).[24] Businesses only pay when internet users clicks on their ad. Most marketing companies and consultants consider both Google Ads and Facebooks Ads to be excellent, cost-effective online advertising options for practices to promote awareness of the business, increase traffic to their websites, and attract new clients. While online advertising can be an effective strategy, it's easy to make mistakes and spend money without a good return on investment. Therefore, many practices find it's beneficial to hire a consultant or marketing company with expertise in digital marketing to help plan and execute online advertising initiatives.

Content marketing refers to creating and sharing relevant, valuable information online to increase brand awareness, attract new customers, and increase business from existing customers.[25] Content marketing is closely related to SEO because original, creative content helps boost the website's ranking in search engine results. Examples of content are blog posts, videos, infographics, case studies, and company stories. The strategy of content marketing is to build trust and rapport with audiences by providing valuable information with the hope that this will ultimately lead to increased sales.

For content marketing to work well, the information shared needs to be unique and personalized. One of the most effective ways to do this is with storytelling. Share stories on the hospital website about the history of the practice, why the practice owner started the business and what they love most about veterinary medicine. People connect to stories much more than facts and statements about what services the hospital provides.

Storytelling can also be used when sharing case studies or successful patient outcomes on social media.

In veterinary medicine, content marketing includes providing educational resources for pet owners. This helps promote veterinarians and their teams as trusted advisors. Educational information is more likely to be read by pet owners if it's highly relevant, engaging, and easy to read. For example, rather than drafting detailed articles on medical topics, have veterinarians write short, timely blog posts on topics of interest to pet owners such as "Three Signs Your Cat May Have Kidney Disease", "Which Plants are Toxic to Your Pet", or "Why Pets Need Dental Care, Too." Include high quality photos with content marketing posts to help grab the reader's attention. Infographics are also an excellent example of visually appealing educational content. An example might be to post the lifecycle of the flea or a chart with pictures of foods that are harmful to pets.

For busy veterinary practice leaders who may not have the time or expertise to devise and execute an effective content marketing strategy, it makes sense to seek outside assistance. There are many companies that help practices create a plan and offer content marketing solutions such as customized copywriting for websites, engaging social media posts, original educational articles, and creative content for blog posts.

Social Media

Having a strong presence on social media is an excellent way to stay connected with pet owners. Facebook is by far the most popular platform so all veterinary practices should have a business Facebook page. Facebook business pages have a variety of features and business tools that includes analytics data, targeted advertising, and call to action buttons such as "Contact Us." Other sites to consider are Instagram, Twitter, YouTube, and LinkedIn. Multiple surveys show younger generations favor social media platforms other than just Facebook. A 2019 survey of millennials and Gen Z found the social media platform with the greatest reach for these two generations was YouTube at over 90% and that Instagram reach was similar to Facebook for both men and women at 69% and 79% respectively.[26]

Social media can be used to provide educational content, practice updates, and relevant notifications to clients. But the real power of social media is its ability to allow the practice to create emotional connections with pet owners and create a sense of community which helps to build client loyalty. To accomplish this goal, aim to post, on average, three times a week.

The key to a successful social media strategy is to consistently interact with people. Posts that share scientific articles or statistics may have valuable information but don't tend to engage followers. When sharing this content, include personal messages about why the information is relevant. Here are ways to enhance content shared on social media:

- Tell stories about the hospital, team members, clients, and patients. Stories are one of the best ways to capture attention and make connections. Stories are also a way to share and celebrate the good work of the hospital. Remember to always get permission to share client and patient information and photos.
- Post photos that show the human-animal bond or photos of the team working. Photos taken at the hospital are more personal and interesting than sharing funny or cute images that may be seen everywhere.
- Post personalized videos such as doctors sharing educational messages or relevant news. These videos don't have to be done professionally but they should be clear and preferably no longer than 3 minutes since people have short attention spans. An excellent example of this type of video happened during the COVID-19 pandemic when practice owners turned to social media to post messages reassuring pet owners their hospital was open for business and offering curbside care to keep everyone safe.
- Ask pet owners questions to encourage dialogue. Examples of engaging questions include "How did you come up with your pet's name?" and "What 3 words best describe your pet?"
- Keep track of which posts result in the most comments and shares, not just likes. These are the kind of posts that will continue to garner attention.

Online Reputation Management

Online reputation management (ORM) is the process of influencing and controlling the business's reputation on the internet. Monitor the business's online presence to ensure it has a positive brand identity on the internet. Not only is it important for the practice's website to show up on the first page of search results, it's critical that pet owners see positive reviews. People pay attention to reviews and may be reluctant to choose a hospital with a rating of less than 4.5 out of 5 or one with multiple negative reviews that cite similar grievances. In addition to enhancing the hospital's image, it has been well documented that positive Google reviews do help improve search rankings and SEO efforts.[27]

Routinely examine online reviews of the business on all sites such as Google, Facebook, and Yelp. One way to do this is to set up notifications in the account for when a new review is posted. Someone on the team should respond to all positive reviews as quickly as possible. Thank clients for their kind words, tell them how happy you are they had an excellent experience, and that you appreciate the opportunity to care for their pet. You can also add a compliment about their pet being careful not to use the name of the pet unless they mentioned it.

Since Google is the most utilized search engine, secure as many positive Google reviews as possible. There are several ways to solicit reviews from clients. One is to make it easy for people to leave reviews by sending automated surveys and review requests via email or text. Another is to simply ask clients who are happy with their experience to share their thoughts online. Doctors and team members alike can say "Ms. Marshall, I'm so glad to hear you're happy with your experiences at our hospital. We love caring for Sophie. We'd appreciate you sharing your positive feedback on Google since many pet owners decide where to bring their pets based on reviews."

Responses to negative reviews can be more challenging. Ideally, keep several stock responses on file that can be edited as appropriate for the review. Having a list of appropriate phrases to pull from saves time and provides the peace of mind of knowing you're prepared to respond when the need arises. (See textbox, "Best practices for Responding to Negative Online Reviews From Clients.")

BEST PRACTICES FOR RESPONDING TO NEGATIVE ONLINE REVIEWS FROM CLIENTS:

- Check the pet's medical record for details and reach out to the client with a phone call to see if they're willing to talk about their concern.
- Online responses should be brief and avoid getting into an argument.
- Make sure responses convey compassion and invite the client to call a specific person at the practice who can help them with their concerns (E.g., "We're sorry to hear you didn't have a good experience at our hospital. We value you as a client and strive to provide high-quality care to you and your pet. Please call (specific name) at 123-444-5678 so we can discuss your concerns.")
- If the client is known to be volatile or irrational and/or the negative review is clearly unreasonable, accusatory, and inflammatory it makes sense to NOT respond as this will likely escalate the situation.
- You can flag reviews that are inappropriate on Google to see if they will remove the review. After claiming your business listing on Yelp, you can dispute a review and request they remove the review.[28]

References

Chapter 1

1. Staver, Mike. 2012. *Leadership Isn't For Cowards*. Hoboken: John Wiley & Sons, Inc.
2. Covey, Stephen R. 1989. *The 7 Habits of Highly Successful People*. New York: Simon & Schuster, Inc.
3. Mindtools. n.d. "Active Listening." Accessed July 9, 2020. https://www.mindtools.com/CommSkll/ActiveListening.htm.
4. Brown, Brene. 2018. *Dare to Lead*. New York: Random House.
5. Thomas J. Zuber, MD, and Erika H. James, PHD. 2001. "Managing Your Boss." Family Practice Management. (June): 33. https://www.aafp.org/fpm/2001/0600/p33.html."
6. Rousmaniere, Dana. 2015. "What Everyone Should Know About Managing Up." January 23, 2015. https://hbr.org/2015/01/what-everyone-should-know-about-managing-up.
7. Kreitner, Robert. 2001. Management. Boston: Houghton Mifflin Company.
8. Kreitner, Robert. 2001. Management. Boston: Houghton Mifflin Company.
9. Horsager, David. 2020. "The Trust Outlook." https://trustedge.com/the-research?s2-ssl=yes.
10. Gallup. n.d. Accessed July 9, 2020. https://www.gallup.com/cliftonstrengths/en/252137/home.aspx.
11. Judgement Index. n.d. "Leadership and Team Development." Accessed July 9, 2020. https://judgmentindex.com/leadership-and-team-development/.
12. AVMA. n.d. Accessed July 9, 2020. https://www.avma.org/.
13. AAHA. n.d. Accessed July 9, 2020. https://www.aaha.org/.
14. VHMA. n.d. Accessed July 9, 2020. https://www.vhma.org/.
15. SHRM. n.d. Accessed July 9, 2020. https://www.shrm.org/resourcesandtools/.

Chapter 2

1. Hill, Charles W.L. and Gareth R. Jones. 2004. *Strategic Management Theory*. Sixth Ed. Boston: Houghton Mifflin Company.
2. Hill, Charles W.L. and, Gareth R. Jones. 2004. *Strategic Management Theory*. Sixth Ed. Boston: Houghton Mifflin Company.
3. SHRM. 2018. "Mission & Vision Statements: What is the difference between mission, vision and values statements?" March 5, 2018. https://www.shrm.org/resourcesandtools/tools-and-samples/hr-qa/pages/isthereadifferencebetweenacompany%E2%80%99smission,visionandvaluestatements.aspx.
4. Mayo Clinic Health System. n.d. "Mission, Vision and Value Statements." Accessed July 14, 2020. https://www.mayoclinichealthsystem.org/locations/eau-claire/about-us/mission-vision-and-value-statements/.
5. Southwest. n.d. *"Southwest Careers"*. Accessed May 2, 2021. https://careers.southwestair.com/culturetemplate.
6. Mayo Clinic Health System. n.d. "Mission, Vision and Value Statements." Accessed July 14, 2020. https://www.mayoclinichealthsystem.org/locations/eau-claire/about-us/mission-vision-and-value-statements/.
7. SHRM. 2018. "What Does it Mean to be a Values-based Organization?" March 8, 2018.

8. Hsieh, Tony. 2010. *Delivering Happiness.* New York, NY: Business Plus.
9. Merriam Webster. n.d. "Professionalism." Accessed July 16, 2020. https://www.merriam-webster.com/dictionary/professionalism.
10. Thompson, Leigh L. 2000. *Making the Team: A Guide for Managers.* Upper Saddle River, NJ: Prentice Hall.
11. Lencioni, Patrick. 2002. *The Five Dysfunctions of A Team.* San Francisco, CA: Jossey-Bass.
12. SHRM. n.d. "Diversity Policy." Accessed July 17, 2020. https://www.shrm.org/resourcesandtools/tools-and-samples/policies/pages/diversitypolicy.aspx?_ga=2.209409627.831554934.1594933004-1908819276.1592946320.
13. Ella Washington, Camille Patrick. 2018. "3 Requirements for a Diverse and Inclusive Culture. "September 17, 2018. https://www.gallup.com/workplace/242138/requirements-diverse-inclusive-culture.aspx.
14. DataUSA. n.d. "Data USA: Veterinarians." Accessed May 2, 2021. https://datausa.io/profile/soc/veterinarians#about.
15. PrideVMC. n.d. *"PrideVMC."* Accessed July 20, 2020. https://pridevmc.org/.
16. Camille Parker and Ella Washington. 2018. "3 Ways Millennials Can Advance Workplace Diversity and Inclusion." November 30, 2018. https://www.gallup.com/workplace/245084/ways-millennials-advance-workplace-diversity-inclusion.aspx.
17. Vanderbilt. n.d. "Equity, Diversity and Inclusion." Accessed July 20, 2020. https://www.vanderbilt.edu/diversity/unconscious-bias/#:~:text=Unconscious%20bias%20(or%20implicit%20bias,that%20is%20usually%20considered%20unfair.
18. Perera, Ayesh. 2021 *"Why the Halo Effect Affects How We Perceive Others."* March 22 2021. https://www.simplypsychology.org/halo-effect.html.
19. Gassam, Janice. 2020. "Are Job Candidates Still Being Penalized For Having 'Ghetto' Names? "February 20, 2020. https://www.forbes.com/sites/janicegassam/2020/02/20/are-job-candidates-still-being-penalized-for-having-ghetto-names/#6e9f2cc550ed.
20. Project Implicit n.d.. Accessed July 20, 2020. https://implicit.harvard.edu/implicit/takeatest.html.
21. McWhorter, John. 2020. "The Dictionary Definition of Racism Has to Change." June 22, 2020. https://www.theatlantic.com/ideas/archive/2020/06/dictionary-definition-racism-has-change/613324/.
22. Merriam Webster. n.d. "Merriam-Webster Micro-Agression." Accessed July 20, 2020. https://www.merriam-webster.com/dictionary/microaggression.
23. Sarkis, Stephanie. 2020. "Let's Talk About Racial Microaggressions In The Workplace." June 15, 2020. https://www.forbes.com/sites/stephaniesarkis/2020/06/15/lets-talk-about-racial-microaggressions-in-the-workplace/#29c3e145d283.
24. Greenhill, Lisa. 2020. "The problem with tone policing." Today's Veterinary Business, April/May: 43-45.
25. Yuan, Karen. 2020. "Black employees say 'performative allyship' is an unchecked problem in the office." June 19, 2020. https://fortune.com/2020/06/19/performative-allyship-working-while-black-white-allies-corporate-diversity-racism/.
26. Lester, Jennifer Mencl and Scott W. 2014. "More Alike Than Different: What Generations Value and How the Values Affect Employee Workplace Perceptions." ResearchGate. June,

2014. https://www.researchgate.net/publication/275475387_More_Alike_Than_Different_What_Generations_Value_and_How_the_Values_Affect_Employee_Workplace_Perceptions.
27. Tomasi, Suzanne E., Ethan D. Fechter-Leggett, Nicole T. Edwards, Anna D. Reddish, Alex E. Crosby, Randall J. Nett. 2019. "Suicide among veterinarians in the United States from 1979 through 2015." (AVMA) 254 (1): 104-112.

Chapter 3

1. Larkin, Malinda. 2019. "Not too much, not too little: Veterinarians try to find sweet spot on hours worked." November 25, 2019. https://www.avma.org/javma-news/2019-12-15/not-too-much-not-too-little-veterinarians-try-find-sweet-spot-hours-worked.
2. Nolen, Scott. 2020. "Veterinary Labor Demand Remains Strong During COVID." JAVMA. January 5, 2021.257: 1214.
3. Larkin, Malinda. 2019. "Technician shortage may be a problem of turnover instead." September 28, 2019. https://www.avma.org/javma-news/2016-10-15/technician-shortage-may-be-problem-turnover-instead.
4. Mattson, Kaitlyn. 2020. *"NAVTA's Veterinary Nurse Initiative a work in progress."* February 26, 2020. https://www.avma.org/javma-news/2020-03-15/navtas-veterinary-nurse-initiative-work-progress.
5. AAHA. 2019. *Financial and Productivity Pulsepoints.* Lakewood: AAHA Press. Accessed August 4, 2020.
6. Tumblin, Denise. 2019. *2019 Well-Managed Practice® Benchmarks Study.* WMPB, LCC. Accessed July 30, 2020.
7. AAHA. 2019. *Financial and Productivity Pulsepoints.* Tenth. Lakewood: AAHA Press. Accessed July 30, 2020.
8. Bain, Bridgette. 2020. "Employment, starting salaries, and educational indebtedness of year-2019 graduates of US veterinary medical colleges." JAVMA August 1, 2020. 257: 296.
9. Great Place to Work. 2019. "Hilton Named the No. 1 Workplace on 2019 Fortune 100 Best Companies to Work For List." February 14, 2019. https://www.prnewswire.com/news-releases/hilton-named-the-no-1-workplace-on-2019-fortune-100-best-companies-to-work-for-list-300795562.html.
10. AAHA. n.d. "Mentorship Accreditation." Accessed July 31, 2020. https://www.aaha.org/accreditation--membership/accreditation-process/mentorship-accreditation/.
11. Cotner, Jennifer R. 2017. "Top 10 Mistakes Employers Make in Job Applications." June 6, 2017. https://www.shrm.org/resourcesandtools/hr-topics/talent-acquisition/pages/top-10-mistakes-employers-make-job-applications.aspx.

Chapter 4

1. Bauer, Talya N. 2010. "Onboarding New Employees: Maximizing Success." August 6, 2020. https://www.shrm.org/foundation/ourwork/initiatives/resources-from-past-initiatives/Documents/Onboarding%20New%20Employees.pdf.
2. Edward Lowe Foundation. n.d. "Value of Orientation." Accessed August 6, 2020. https://edwardlowe.org/value-of-orientation/#:~:text=Often%2C%20an%20employee%20will%20

3. Maurer, Rob. n.d. "New Employee Onboarding Guide." Accessed August 10, 2020. https://shrm.org/resourcesandtools/hr-topics/talent-acquisition/pages/new-employee-onboarding-guide.aspx?_ga=2.98679454.1873684981.1596647632-1908819276.1592946320.
4. Mindtools. n.d. "VAK Learning Styles." Accessed August 13, 2020. https://www.mindtools.com/pages/article/vak-learning-styles.htm.
5. Willingham, Daniel T. 2018. "Ask the Cognitive Scientist: Does Tailoring Instruction to "Learning Styles" Help Students Learn?" https://www.aft.org/ae/summer2018/willingham.
6. Gurchiek, Kathy. 2017. "Considering Reverse Mentoring? Check Out These Tips." November 10, 2017. https://www.shrm.org/resourcesandtools/hr-topics/organizational-and-employee-development/pages/considering-reverse-mentoring-check-out-these-tips.aspx.

Chapter 5

1. Lloyd, Sam. n.d. "Managers Must Delegate Effectively to Develop Employees." Accessed August 19, 2020. https://www.shrm.org/resourcesandtools/hr-topics/organizational-and-employee-development/pages/delegateeffectively.aspx#:~:text=Often%2C%20managers%20think%20that%20they,to%20produce%20the%20desired%20results.
2. Ben Wigert and Ryan Pendell. 2020. "The Ultimate Guide to Micromanagers: Signs, Causes, Solutions." July 17, 2020. https://www.gallup.com/workplace/315530/ultimate-guide-micromanagers-signs-causes-solutions.aspx.
3. Schwarz, Roger. 2013. "The Sandwich Approach Undermines Your Feedback." Harvard Business Review. April 19, 2013. https://hbr.org/2013/04/the-sandwich-approach-undermin.
4. Musser, Chris. 2019. "Give Employees the Right Kind of Feedback at the Right Time." December 6, 2019. https://www.gallup.com/workplace/268937/give-employees-right-kind-feedback-right-time.aspx?version=print.
5. Halvorson, Heidi Grant. 2012. *Succeed.* New York: Penguin Group.
6. Halvorson, Heidi Grant. 2012. *Succeed.* New York: Penguin Group.
7. Wakeman, Cy. 2017. *No Ego.* New York: St. Martin's Press.
8. Paychex. 2019. "HR Compliance: What Business Owners Need to Know." April 26, 2019. https://www.paychex.com/articles/human-resources/balance-hr-strategy-compliance#:~:text=HR%20compliance%20is%20a%20process,larger%20human%20capital%20resources%20objectives.
9. U.S. Equal Employment Opportunity Commission. n.d. "How can I avoid breaking the law when I discipline or fire an employee?" Accessed August 27, 2020. https://www.eeoc.gov/employers/small-business/7-how-can-i-avoid-breaking-law-when-i-discipline-or-fire-employee.
10. Howard, Eric. 2019. "Are You Making These Performance Review Mistakes?" February 7, 2019. https://www.employmentlawhandbook.com/human-resources/are-you-making-these-performance-review-mistakes/.
11. Lizotte, Jaimie. 2018. "Correct and Protect: Your Guide to Employee Discipline and Termination." March 5, 2018. https://www.hrdirectapps.com/blog/your-guide-to-employee-discipline-and-termination/.
12. Nagele-Piazza, Lisa. 2018. "12 Tips for Handling Employee Terminations and Disciplinary Actions." March 15, 2018. https://shrm.org/resourcesandtools/legal-and-

compliance/employment-law/pages/12-tips-for-handling-employee-terminations.aspx?_ga=2.247775367.1280369552.1598456079-1908819276.1592946320.

13. Lizotte, Jaimie. 2018. "Correct and Protect: Your Guide to Employee Discipline and Termination." March 5, 2018. https://www.hrdirectapps.com/blog/your-guide-to-employee-discipline-and-termination/.
14. Guerin, Lisa. 2015. "Legal Issues to Consider When Disciplining Employees." April 9, 2015. https://www.lawyers.com/legal-info/labor-employment-law/human-resources-law/employers-must-follow-employee-discipline-procedures.html.
15. Comply Right. 2019. "State Leave Laws: What You Need to Know." February 1, 2019. https://www.complyright.com/employee-leave/what-you-need-to-know-about-state-leave-laws.
16. Taylor, Steve. 2011. "Assess Pros and Cons of 360-Degree Performance Appraisal." July 12, 2011. https://www.shrm.org/resourcesandtools/hr-topics/employee-relations/pages/360degreeperformance.aspx.
17. SHRM. n.d. "How to Establish a Performance Improvement Plan." Accessed September 14, 2020. https://www.shrm.org/resourcesandtools/tools-and-samples/how-to-guides/pages/performanceimprovementplan.aspx.

Chapter 6

1. Indeed. n.d. "Calculating Retention Rate: A Guide for Managers." Accessed October 1, 2020. https://www.indeed.com/hire/c/info/calculate-retention-rate?aceid=&gclid=EAIaIQobChMI6YWW7a-U7AIVFYzICh22bgVfEAAYAiAAEgLA2fD_BwE.
2. Gallup. n.d. "What Is Employee Engagement and How Do You Improve It?" Accessed October 5, 2020. https://www.gallup.com/workplace/285674/improve-employee-engagement-workplace.aspx#:~:text=Gallup%20defines%20engaged%20employees%20as,to%20their%20work%20and%20workplace.
3. SHRM. n.d. "Managing Employee Surveys." Accessed October 5, 2020. https://www.shrm.org/resourcesandtools/tools-and-samples/toolkits/pages/managingemployeesurveys.aspx.
4. Gallup. n.d. "What Is Employee Engagement and How Do You Improve It?" Accessed October 5, 2020. https://www.gallup.com/workplace/285674/improve-employee-engagement-workplace.aspx#:~:text=Gallup%20defines%20engaged%20employees%20as,to%20their%20work%20and%20workplace.
5. HR Technologist. 2019. "Pulse Surveys vs. Annual Surveys: Which Is a Better Measure of Employee Engagement?" May 17, 2019. https://www.hrtechnologist.com/articles/employee-engagement/pulse-surveys-vs-annual-surveys-which-is-a-better-measure-of-employee-engagement/.
6. Engage Employee. 2020. "Ditch the 'Exit' Interview for the 'Stay' Interview." August 12, 2020. https://engageemployee.com/ditch-the-exit-interview-for-the-stay-interview/.
7. SHRM. n.d. "Stay Interview Questions." https://www.shrm.org/resourcesandtools/tools-and-samples/hr-forms/pages/stayinterviewquestions.aspx.
8. Indeed. 2020. "Intrinsic Rewards: What They Are and Why They're Important". January 3, 2020. https://www.indeed.com/career-advice/career-development/intrinsic-rewards.
9. Thomas, Kenneth. 2009. "The Four Intrinsic Rewards that Drive Employee Engagement." November/December 2009. https://iveybusinessjournal.com/publication/

Leading and Managing Veterinary Teams

10. Harter, James A., Frank L. Schmidt, Sangeeta Agrawal, Anthony Blue, Stephanie K. Plowman, Patrick Josh, Jim Asplund. 2020. "The Powerful Relationship Between Employee Engagement and Team Performance." Gallup. October 2020. https://www.gallup.com/workplace/321032/employee-engagement-meta-analysis-brief.aspx.
11. SHTM. 2016. "Employee Job Satisfaction and Engagement: Revitalizing a Changing Workforce." April 18, 2016. https://www.shrm.org/hr-today/trends-and-forecasting/research-and-surveys/pages/job-satisfaction-and-engagement-report-revitalizing-changing-workforce.aspx.
12. Robbins, Mike. 2019. "Why Employees Need Both Recognition and Appreciation." November 12, 2019. https://hbr.org/2019/11/why-employees-need-both-recognition-and-appreciation.
13. Horsager, David. 2018. "The Trust Outlook." Trust Edge Leadership Institute. https://trustedge.com/the-research?s2-ssl=yes.
14. O'Boyle, Ed. 2021. "4 Things Gen Z and Millennials Expect From Their Workplace." March 30, 2021. https://www.gallup.com/workplace/336275/things-gen-millennials-expect-workplace.aspx?utm_source=workplace&utm_medium=email&utm_campaign=workplace_newsletter_apr_04062021&utm_term=newsletter&utm_content=four_things_textlink_1&elqTrackId=330cea48a09a4ef487b.
15. Dimock, Michael. 2019. "Defining generations: Where Millennials end and Generation Z begins." January 17, 2019. https://www.pewresearch.org/fact-tank/2019/01/17/where-millennials-end-and-generation-z-begins/.
16. O'Boyle, Ed. 2021. "4 Things Gen Z and Millennials Expect From Their Workplace." March 30, 2021. https://www.gallup.com/workplace/336275/things-gen-millennials-expect-workplace.aspx?utm_source=workplace&utm_medium=email&utm_campaign=workplace_newsletter_apr_04062021&utm_term=newsletter&utm_content=four_things_textlink_1&elqTrackId=330cea48a09a4ef487b.
17. Robison, Jenny. 2019. "Why Millennials Are Job Hopping." October 28, 2019. https://www.gallup.com/workplace/267743/why-millennials-job-hopping.aspx.
18. Stillman, David Stillman and Jonah. 2017. "Move Over, Millennials; Generation Z Is Here." April 11, 2017. https://www.shrm.org/resourcesandtools/hr-topics/behavioral-competencies/global-and-cultural-effectiveness/pages/move-over-millennials-generation-z-is-here.aspx.
19. AVMA. 2020. "Task force recommends solutions for technician utilization." https://www.avma.org/javma-news/task-force-recommends-solutions-technician-utilization.
20. Cambridge Dictionary. n.d. "Meaning of team building." Accessed October 7, 2020. https://dictionary.cambridge.org/us/dictionary/english/team-building.

Chapter 7

1. Lindsay MacGregor and Neel Doshi. 2015. "Let Science Explain Why Your Co-workers are Slackers." December 4, 2015. https://www.fastcompany.com/3054170/the-scientific-reason-why-some-people-are-slackers.
2. Lexico. n.d. "Passive agressive." Accessed October 30, 2020. https://www.lexico.com/en/definition/passive-aggressive.

3. Bahl, Meghna. 2010. "Identify and Respond to Passive Aggression at Work." October 29, 2010. https://www.shrm.org/resourcesandtools/hr-topics/employee-relations/pages/passiveaggressionatwork.aspx.
4. Mindtools. n.d. "How to Manage Passive-Aggressive People." Accessed October 30, 2020. https://www.mindtools.com/pages/article/passive-aggressive-people.htm.
5. Wilkie, Dana. n.d. "Workplace Gossip: What Crosses the Line?" Accessed November 2, 2020. https://www.shrm.org/resourcesandtools/hr-topics/employee-relations/pages/office-gossip-policies.aspx.
6. Inc. 2020. "Employee Motivation." February 6, 2020. https://www.inc.com/encyclopedia/employee-motivation.html.
7. Fowler, Susan. 2014. *Why Motivating People Doesn't Work…and What Does*. San Francisco: Berrett-Koehler Publishers, Inc.
8. Browning, Michelle. 2018. "Self-Leadership: Why It Matters." International Journal of Business and Social Science 9 (2): 14-18. https://ijbssnet.com/journals/Vol_9_No_2_February_2018/2.pdf.
9. Ken Blanchard, Susan Fowler, Laurence Hawkins. 2017. *Self Leadership and the One Minute Manager*. William Morrow.

Chapter 8

1. Walsh, Sandy. 2018. "The efficient practice." February 2018. https://todaysveterinarybusiness.com/the-efficient-practice/.
2. Shupe, Christine. 2015. "What's standard for veterinary medical standards?" December 15, 2015. https://www.dvm360.com/view/whats-standard-veterinary-medical-standards.

Chapter 9

1. Lexico. n.d. "Key performance indicator." Accessed May 2, 2021. https://www.lexico.com/definition/key_performance_indicator.
2. Merriam Webster. n.d. "Benchmark." Accessed July 2, 2020. https://www.merriam-webster.com/dictionary/benchmark.
3. Vetsuccess. 2020. "AVMA chief economist weighs in on recent findings: Veterinary ACT versus visits for revenue". July 7, 2020. https://vetsuccess.com/blog/veterinary-act-versus-visits-for-revenue/.
4. Lowell Ackerman, DVM, DACVD, MBA, MPA, CVA, MRCVS. 2020. "Making Valid Comparisons Between Practices and Services." In *Blackwell's Five-Minute Veterinary Practice Management Consult*. 466-467. Hoboken: Wiley Blackwell.
5. Salois, Matthew. 2021. "Are we in a veterinary workforce crisis?" 2021. https://www.avma.org/javma-news/2021-09-15/are-we-veterinary-workforce-crisis.
6. AAHA. 2019. *Financial and Productivity Pulsepoints*. Tenth Ed. Lakewood: AAHA Press.
7. Tumblin, Denise, Tassava, Brenda. 2019. 2019 Well-Managed Practice® Benchmarks Study.
8. Felsted, Karen. 2020. VHMA Insider's Insights. Alachua, FL. Accessed July 8, 2020.
9. American Heartworm Society. n.d. "Heartworm Guidelines." Accessed July 8, 2020. https://www.heartwormsociety.org/index.php.
10. AAHA. n.d. "Chart of Accounts." Accessed July 8, 2020. https://www.aaha.org/

practice-resources/running-your-practice/chart-of-accounts/.
11. Mark Opperman, CVPM. 2019. "Pro on Pro-Sal." February 2019. https://todaysveterinary-business.com/pro-on-prosal/.
12. AAHA. 2018. *The Veterinary Fee Reference.* Tenth Ed. Lakewood, CO: AAHA Press.
13. VetPartners. n.d. "Practice Valuation Resources." Accessed July 9, 2020. https://www.vet-partners.org/practice-valuation-resources/.

Chapter 10

1. American Marking Association. n.d. Accessed July 9, 2020. https://www.ama.org/the-definition-of-marketing-what-is-marketing/.
2. Mindtools. n.d. "Smart Goals." Accessed July 9, 2020. https://www.mindtools.com/pages/article/smart-goals.htm.
3. Fleming, John H and Jim Asplund. 2007. *Human Sigma.* New York: Gallup Press.
4. Gallup. 2006. "Nurses Top List of Most Honest and Ethical Professions." December 14, 2006. https://news.gallup.com/poll/25888/nurses-top-list-most-honest-ethical-professions.aspx.
5. Shaw Jane R. 2006. "Four Core Communication Skills of Highly Effective Practitioners." *Veterinary Clinics Small Animal Practice.* Philadelphia: Elsevier Saunders.
6. Silverman, Jonathan, Suzanne Kurtz, Juliet Draper. 2005. *Skills for Communicating with Patients.* Oxford: Radcliffe Publishing.
7. YouTube. n.d. "Brené Brown on Empathy." Accessed July 9, 2020. https://www.youtube.com/watch?v=1Evwgu369Jw.
8. Alina M. Kuper and Roswitha Merle. 2019. "Being Nice Is Not Enough-Exploring Relationship-Centered Veterinary Care With Structural Equation Modeling. A Quantitative Study on German Pet Owners' Perception." February 28, 2019. https://www.ncbi.nlm.nih.gov/pmc/articles/PMC6403131/.
9. Ackerman, Lowell. 2021. *Pet Specific Care for the Veterinary Teams.* Hoboken, NJ: John Wiley & Sons, Inc.
10. Ackerman, Lowell. 2018. "An Introduction to Pet-Specific Care." December 9, 2018. http://balkanvets.com/index.php/2018/12/09/an-introduction-to-pet-specific-care/.
11. Gutierrez, K. 2014. "Studies Confirm the Power of Visuals to Engage Your Audience in E-Learning." July 10, 2014. https://www.shiftelearning.com/blog/bid/350326/studies-confirm-the-power-of-visuals-in-elearning.
12. AAHA. 2003. "The Path to High-Quality Care: Practical Tips For Improving Compliance." Lakewood: AAHA Press.
13. AAHA. 2009. "Compliance follow-up study." Lakewood: AAHA Press.
14. McReynolds, Tony. 2019. "Heartworm compliance study: Just because you're sick of talking about heartworm prevention doesn't mean your clients are." May 2, 2019. https://www.aaha.org/publications/newstat/articles/2019-05/heartworm-compliance-study-just-because-youre-sick-of-talking-about-heartworm-prevention-doesnt-mean-your-clients-are/.
15. Volk, John O., Karen E. Felsted, James G. Thomas, Colin W Siren. 2011. "Executive summary of the Bayer Veterinary Care Usage Study." JAVMA, 238, 1275-1282.
16. Kanji, Noureen, Jason B. Coe, Cindy L. Adams, Jane R. Shaw. 2012. "Effect of

References

veterinarian-client-patient interactions on client adherence to dentistry and surgery recommendations in companion-animal practice." JAVMA, 240, 427-434.
17. AVMA. 2018. AVMA Pet Owner and Demographics Sourcebook. https://www.avma.org.
18. Banfield. 2015. https://www.banfield.com/veterinary-professionals/resources/soph-infographic.
19. AVMA. n.d. Accessed July 9, 2020. https://www.avma.org/resources-tools/avma-policies/human-animal-interaction-and-human-animal-bond.).
20. Fry, Richard. 2020. "Millennials overtake Baby Boomers as America's largest generation." April 28, 2020. https://www.pewresearch.org/fact-tank/2020/04/28/millennials-overtake-baby-boomers-as-americas-largest-generation/.
21. Vogels, E. A. 2019. "Millennials stand out for their technology use, but older generations also embrace digital life." September 19, 2019. https://www.pewresearch.org/fact-tank/2019/09/09/us-generations-technology-use/.
22. Hyken, Shep. 2018. *The Convenience Revolution*. Shippensburg: Sound Wisdom.
23. Alexander, Lucy. 2021. "The Who, What, Why, & How of Digital Marketing." Updated October 7, 2021. https://blog.hubspot.com/marketing/what-is-digital-marketing.
24. WordStream. n.d. "Facebook Ads vs. Google AdWords: Which Should You Be Using?" Accessed July 2020. https://www.wordstream.com/facebook-vs-google.
25. Miller, Jason. 2016. "What Is Content Marketing? Definitions from 25 Thought Leaders." February 2, 2016. https://business.linkedin.com/marketing-solutions/blog/best-practices--content-marketing/2016/what-is-content-marketing--definitions-from-25-thought-leaders.
26. Tankovska, H. 2021.). "Reach of selected social media platforms among Gen Z and Millennial internet users in the United States as of September 2019, by gender." January 28, 2021. https://www.statista.com/statistics/471543/millennials-usa-social-media-reach-gender/.
27. Kehoe, Bob. n.d. "Do Google Reviews Help Rankings and SEO?" Accessed July 9, 2020. https://www.theleverageway.com/blog/do-google-reviews-help-rankings-seo/.
28. Garcia, Eric. 2018. "Turn a Negative into a Positive." December 2018. https://todaysveterinarybusiness.com/turn-a-negative-into-a-positive/.

APPENDIX A

Detailed Table of Contents

1 Becoming a Successful Manager

Defining Success

Being Proactive Vs. Reactive

Establishing Job Expectations

Enhancing Productivity

Honing Communication Skills
- Active listening
- Transparent communication
- Asking good questions
- Setting boundaries

Managing Up

Leadership Development
- Leadership roles and building trust:
  - Clarity
  - Competency
  - Compassion
  - Consistency
- Identify strengths and weaknesses
- Personality testing and assessment tools
- Professional development

2 Enhancing the Hospital Culture

Strategic Planning:
- Developing mission and vision
- SWOT analysis

- Setting business goals

Establishing Core Values
- What is a core value?
- Helping teams understand your core values

Making Your Desired Culture a Reality
- Create a values-based culture
- Professionalism
- Encouraging teamwork

Promoting Diversity and Inclusion
- Overcoming unconscious bias
- Committing to anti-racism
- Celebrating employee differences

Work-life Balance and Well-being
- Work-life strategies for managers
- Promoting a culture of work-life balance
- Enhancing team well-being

3 Recruiting and Hiring Team Members

Defining Your Ideal Candidate

Compensation and Benefits

Effective Ads
- Where to place ads
- Choose the right words

Becoming a Preferred Employer
- Building the hospital reputation
- Increasing awareness

Conducting Effective Interviews
- Screening candidates
- Avoiding discrimination

- Asking effective questions

Evaluating candidates and making Job Offers

4 Team Training

Employee Orientation

Successfully On-boarding New Hires

Setting Up Effective Training Programs
- How to handle time constraints
- Resources for training
- Learning styles

Leadership Training for Middle Managers

5 Enhancing and Evaluating Job Performance

Managing By Core Values

Effective Delegation
- Defining job duties, roles, and expectations
- Oversight vs. micro-management

Feedback
- How to give meaningful feedback
- Giving negative feedback positively

Accountability
- Identifying causes of lack of accountability
- Holding effective accountability meetings

Legal Issues
- Avoiding discrimination
- Documentation
- Compliance with laws

Conducting Performance Reviews

- Develop a consistent process
- Communication Best Practices

Discipline And Performance Improvement Plans
- Progressive discipline
- How to write an effective PIP

Termination

6 Employee Retention

Understanding Employee Engagement
- Engagement surveys
- Exit surveys and stay interviews
- Extrinsic vs. intrinsic rewards

Employee Engagement Strategies
- Enhancing employee-manager relationships
- Building trust with the team
- Consider generational differences
- Employee development
- Technician utilization
- Employee empowerment

Team Building

7 Communication Challenges and Solutions

Handling Difficult Employees
- Understanding behavior and managing conversations
- Dealing with problem behaviors
  - Poor work ethic and apathy
  - Negativity
  - Passive aggression

Detailed Table of Contents

- Gossip and unprofessional behavior

Conflict Resolution
- Strategies to prevent employee conflict
- Facilitation of conflict resolution meetings

Employee Motivation and Self-Leadership
- Understanding employee motivation
- How to encourage self-leadership

Helping Employees Embrace Change

8 Hospital Operations

Operational Efficiency
- Processes to improve efficiency
  - Appointment scheduling
  - Patient admission and discharge
  - Exam room flow
  - Leveraging technology
- Implementing protocols and standard operating procedures
  - Establishing protocols and SOPs
  - Setting medical standards

Holding Effective Team Meetings
- Define the purpose and agenda of meetings
- The art of facilitation
- Set deadlines and establish action plans
- Standing meetings and morning huddles

Inventory Management
- Designate an inventory manager
- Determine quantity on hand amounts and reorder points

9 Financial Management

Key Performance Indicators
- Industry benchmarks
- Total revenue
- Income categories
- Number of transactions
- Average transaction charge
- Doctor productivity
  - Revenue production
  - Doctor transactions
  - Average doctor transaction
- Team productivity
- New clients and patients
- Client retention and client visitation
- Active clients and patients
- Client compliance
- Setting goals to improve

Understanding Profit & Loss Statements
- Expense control
  - Facility expenses
  - COGS
  - Staff and doctor payroll

Pricing Strategies
- Market-based pricing
- Cost-based pricing
- Value-based pricing
- Setting fees

Understanding Practice Profitability

10 Marketing and Client Communications

Marketing Strategy
- Evaluate KPIs
- Internal and external marketing
- Focus on target markets

Establishing Marketing goals

Implementing Marketing Plans
- Developing tactics
- Measuring Success

Client Acquisition
- Location and hospital appearance
- Print advertising
- Internet
- Client referrals
- Creating awareness
- Converting phone calls to appointments

Client Engagement
- Building trust
- Core client communication skills
  - Non-verbal communication
  - Open-ended questions
  - Reflective listening
  - Empathy statements

Client Education
- Partnering with clients
- Improving client education messages
- Use of visual tools

Increasing Client Compliance
- Reminder systems
- Communicating value
- Making clear recommendations
- Talking about money
- Forward booking
- Handling angry clients

Building Client Loyalty and Meeting Client's Needs
- Human animal bond
- Generational differences
- Convenient, personalized service
- Client loyalty programs

Digital Marketing
- Websites and search engine optimization
- Ads and content marketing
- Social media
- Online reputation management

About the Author

Dr. Amanda Donnelly is a nationally recognized speaker and consultant specializing in leadership, team development, and client communications. She travels across the U.S. to help veterinarians and managers become better leaders and teach teams how to enhance the client service experience. Dr. Donnelly received her Doctorate in Veterinary Medicine from the University of Missouri and began her professional career with 15 years of clinical experience in small animal practice and emergency medicine in Kansas City. After working four years as a Professional Services Veterinarian in California, she went back to school and earned her MBA prior to founding her consulting and speaking business. Dr. Donnelly is the author and co-author of multiple books and has published numerous articles in veterinary journals. Well known for her dynamic and engaging speaking style, she brings her business knowledge and passion to life for national and international audiences alike. What makes Dr. Donnelly unique is her ability to relate to all members of the team and deliver programs filled with actionable takeaways. Dr. Donnelly lives with her adorable dog in Nashville, Tennessee. When not working, she enjoys outdoor activities, traveling to new destinations, watching football (Go Chiefs and Titans) and spending time with family and friends. She can be emailed at adonnelly@aldvet.com

Made in the USA
Las Vegas, NV
24 August 2023

76550432R00157